Lisa's Counter Culture

Pickles and Other Well-Bred Foods

BY LISA HERNDON

Lisa's Counter Culture
P.O. Box 60696
Palo Alto, CA 94306

Herndon, Lisa
Lisa's Counter Culture: Pickles and Other Well-Bred Foods — 1st ed.

Cover Photo Credit: Adam Silver

Includes index.
LCCN: 2012914448
ISBN-13: 978-0-9858408-0-8

Printed in the USA
www.LisasCounterCulture.com

Table of Contents

Section 2: Ferment Companions

Preface

I'm often asked how I got started fermenting and cooking counter culture foods. My short story: It's been an interestingly crazy and challenging exploration—one that continues to unfold.

First, let me address an important point. I am not a trained chef or a certified nutritionist. I am not a doctor, and I don't give medical advice. So who am I?

I am a concerned mother, wife and fellow human being who cares deeply about nutrition and our environment. I want real food that is nourishing for me, my family and for the world overall. I want to feel confident that I am contributing to life friendly practices that impact our ecosystems like animal husbandry. I have spent the last 10 years consumed with researching and experimenting with traditional food preparation. In particular, I have made many discoveries as I have delved deeper into the biochemistry of fermentation. As a result, I have made adjustments to some of my recipes and techniques. This book reflects what I believe is true and accurate.

I love to teach workshops and share what I have learned. I also love to coach and to assist others to find answers to pesky chronic health problems that much of western medicine is not adept at managing or resolving. I find deep satisfaction in connecting people to resources and healers to aid in their relief of such ailments.

So here's my longer story:

I was fortunate to be exposed to many real foods as a child. Thanks mom! Then our culture began to change when "experts" started claiming that nonfat and seed oil products were best and that raw milk was certainly dangerous. My family, like most others, believed these experts and made changes at home. The change in our milk selection was one of the more dramatic changes that I remember. Another sudden change was the general idea that fats were bad. Skinless chicken breasts started to appear on the dinner table as did diet soda (not for us kids, but for the adults).

As a teenager, I drank a lot of diet soda in order to be "thin." I became a vegetarian to boot. My saving grace was that I continued to eat fish, eggs, and cheese. But still, my health suffered. Mood swings and energy dips were common because of drops in my sugar levels after eating carbohydrate heavy meals. My health got worse as a young adult when I started to cook for myself. I regularly ate low-calorie microwave "meals." And cooking from cans and pre-mixes seemed efficient and economical. (Have you ever noticed the abundance of coupons for processed foods but not many for good, nutritional food?)

Fast forward to my married life. I now had another person to consider when cooking meals. So I started to question the health benefits of these easy-to-cook pre-packaged foods. Then, when I was pregnant with my first child, I became quite nervous and concerned about the little spirit relying on me for nourishment.

I consulted with a nutritionist who recommended *Nourishing Traditions*. This book made a lot of sense to me! But during my two pregnancies, I was diagnosed with gestational diabetes and had to use a blood sugar monitor to watch my sugar levels. I was determined to use diet and exercise to protect my unborn children rather than resorting to medications as a preventive measure. This plan of action worked for me.

I also learned firsthand a lot about how certain foods are digested and how they affect blood sugar levels. I became "Paleo*" without even knowing the term! I was mostly eating protein, fat and non starchy vegetables with just teeny bits of rice or potatoes. I switched from nonfat milk to whole milk and then to raw whole milk. Raw whole milk had the least adverse affect on my blood sugar and caused no "crashing" later either. And amazingly enough, I had a hard time gaining weight, even though I ate fat and protein all the time! Ha! That was a new concept for me. High quality fats did not make me fat!

Rediscovering what past generations have taken for granted has been a blessing and revelation. And having a family and making nutritional decisions about nourishment is a responsibility that I have taken to heart. I continue to fine tune my processes as I learn and discover more about food and how it's grown, raised and prepared for consumption. I hope you are inspired to try some of the ideas and techniques found in this book in your own home.

*My definition of Paleo is a bit more flexible than some others. I believe in eating whole, unprocessed foods with appropriate amounts of dairy or grains, as tolerated by the individual. I don't find Paleo to be a perfect diet for everyone. It needs a bit of tweaking to suit each person individually. If you are happy and healthy with your diet, than I am supportive of what is working for you.

Acknowledgments

I am new to the book writing process, so please forgive me if I have neglected to mention a person or resource that assisted me on my path to completing this book.

I want to first thank my family; my husband, Bruce; and my children, Annika and Branson, for inspiring me to get in the kitchen and figure things out! I also want give them thanks for allowing me the time to focus on finally getting this book completed. They have been my super supportive cheerleaders all the way through.

Next up is my mentor Kathleen Mills, who is the brain behind Pickl-It™. Like her, I was searching for a way to properly ferment food to heal myself and improve the health of my family. I, too, was inspired by the books *Nourishing Traditions* by Sally Fallon and *Wild Fermentation* by Sandor Katz, but found that these recipes for fermentation were not quite right for me or my family. Thankfully, Kathleen steered me to the science behind it all and the means to provide the correct conditions in our modern kitchens to achieve true, traditional probiotic-rich food. Thanks again, Kathleen, for all your wisdom and patience.

I am grateful for the research and information provided by the Weston A. Price Foundation. (Become a member!). Thank you also to Chris Kresser, Robb Wolf and Mark Sisson for being trail-blazers to truly nutrient dense foods.

I would also like to thank my amazing mom, who keeps me balanced by making sure I am not in the red. My professional photographer and web guru, Adam Silver, for making the photos and cover to this book pretty!

Thanks to Rose Dawson for brainstorming my book's subtitle.

And of course, to all the wonderful workshop and coaching clients who provided the kick in the you-know-where to finally get this book done! *Lisa's Counter Culture: Pickles and Other Well Bred Foods* would never have been conceived without you. I hope this book meets your expectations and gets stained and tattered in your kitchens!

Introduction

How To Use This Book

This book has two main sections, **Ferments** and **Ferment Companions**.

Ferments is all about the history, science and the art of homemade ferments. I have included the ferments that I am most familiar with and that I regularly make. There are many more to explore, but the principles you learn here are transferable.

In my opinion, fermented foods serve two main functions. First, they improve the digestibility and absorption of meals. Ideally, eat them along with the foods found in the Ferment Companions section. The second function is that they add flavor and preserve seasonal foods for our enjoyment later.

Ferment Companions is everything else: all the real nutrient-rich foods that we eat along with our ferments. The emphasis is on traditional nutrient dense foods.

All recipes are gluten and soy free (except for "Miso Dressing" on page 83) I try to avoid soy products but I do feel comfortable using small amounts of fermented soy in the form of miso or gluten-free soy sauce.

Ingredients

I encourage you to find the highest quality food possible. Find a farmer's market or a local farmer! Get to know where and how your food is grown. Check **Food Resources** on page 133. Local and sustainable ingredients are usually the tastiest and freshest. The recipes in this book are written with certain specifications. If you carefully follow these guidelines (especially critical in the Ferments section), I am confident that your food preparations will be of the highest probiotic density and taste amazing. I have written these recipes with the following particular assumptions:

<u>Water</u>: A clean source without fluoride, chlorine, and other toxins. Filtered spring water or reverse osmosis water are good options.

<u>Salt</u>: Pure unrefined salt without additives (iodine or anti-caking agents). I recommend Himalayan salt because it is a deep mine salt free of the toxins now commonly found in sea salt. Himalayan salt contains no impurities from environmental pollution. Another issue with sea salt is moisture. Often, it's not dried entirely. Moisture can encourage

mold. Himalayan salt is quite dry and this is not an issue. Himalayan salt has a unique crystalline structure and is revered for its taste and medicinal properties.

Vegetable/Fruit: Pesticide free is essential. Organic is even better. Note that all fruits are vegetables, but not all vegetables are fruit. Fruit is defined as the ovary of the plant—a good clue is the presence of seeds. Seeds present = fruit. Did you know that the tomato, cucumber, zucchini, and pumpkin are all fruits?

Egg: Pastured and organic. Soy and corn-free fed are even better.

Meat: Grassfed for cattle, lamb, goat and other ruminants. Animals should be pastured. Note: pigs and poultry are omnivores so grassfed is not a viable option.

Dairy: Pastured, grassfed, raw and organic are optimum. Read more on choosing milk on page 49.

Fat and Oil: Organic, pastured/grassfed for animal fats. It's important to carefully choose high quality animal fats because fat is where toxins are stored in. Poorly fed and raised animals produce poor fats. It's best to choose a stable oil that will not oxidize or turn rancid in high heat cooking.

- High heat use: Lard, tallow, bacon, duck fat, ghee, and coconut oil.
- Cold use: Organic, extra virgin and cold-pressed forms are ideal. Olive oil, butter, sesame oil, avocado oil, and cold expeller press sunflower oil. This is not an exhaustive list, but it should give you a good range of fats and oils to work with.

Sweetener: Unrefined sugar for ferments. Use honey, unrefined maple syrup or coconut palm sugar for ferment companion recipes. Note that honey is a natural antibacterial.

Meal ideas

There are endless possibilities of how to combine foods to make a meal. Here's what I do. Ideally with each meal, I offer a protein, fat, vegetables/fruit and a ferment. And generally, I offer starches with one or two meals daily.

Dinner is the one meal that we as families almost always eat together. I like the concept of courses, so I always serve them in this order:

1. Protein/fat (e.g., slow roasted baby back ribs)
2. Cooked vegetables (usually cooked with fat/oil) and/or fermented veggies
3. Small portion of starch (if being served)
4. Raw vegetables (usually crudite or a salad)

Here's why I like this order: the most nutrient dense foods are consumed first. Then, the next most digestible part of the meal is served (cooked veggies/ferments), ending with the most difficult to digest—the raw veggies/salad. By the end of the meal, your digestive system is primed with enzymes, and you are less likely to overeat or be too full before getting in those needed fats and proteins. If I offer dessert (mostly for the kids), I serve it a few hours later and right after a cheese/nut (protein/fat) snack. Dessert portions are small and are to be savored.

Required Reading for the Ferments Section!

I must emphasize that it's very important that you read this section before starting a ferment recipe! The following specific points apply to all the ferment recipes included in this book. Please be sure to take the time to carefully read this section.

The benefits of fermented foods

Because you are made mostly of bacteria and there is a constant battle of good versus bad bacteria, ferments give you an edge over the bad by repopulating the good flora into your body. At least 70% of your body's immune function is a result of a healthy gastrointestinal tract. But we often tax our systems with antibiotics, processed foods, chronic stress, dietary toxins (like wheat and seed oils), and numerous other factors that deplete our body's immune function. That's why fermented foods are so beneficial in restoring gut health.

Living fermented foods are likely more effective than probiotic supplements. Supplements must undergo a vigorous manufacturing process, so there is no guarantee that the beneficial bacteria will survive before you get them into your system. Living ferments are powerful so start slowly and with small amounts to avoid die off (page 18).

It's easy to incorporate ferments into your daily routine. Condiments like fermented mayonnaise, chutneys, salsas and krauts are easy to prepare and simple to add to meals. Fermented beverages are a delicious low or no sugar addition. My family loves having kombucha, fermented lemonade, or beet kvass with our meals.

I hope that I have inspired you to add fermented foods to your daily diet. I find that they make our meals more enjoyable and reduce the cravings for carbohydrates and sugar. You will also discover that young children do enjoy tangy fermented foods. I have enjoyed watching children who for the first time taste fermented green beans, carrots or even pickle kraut and request more. This makes my heart swell!

Fermentation versus pickling

A common misconception about fermentation is that it is pickling. Initially, this term was more accurate. But now, most "pickled" products are made with vinegar and heated at high heat to preserve them. I refer to these foods as jarred foods. These are commonly found on the unrefrigerated shelves at your grocer or from someone "canning" at home to preserve vegetables such as carrots, sauerkraut, jams, etc. This is a way to preserve food. However, a big drawback is that they often have preservatives added and the live enzymes are killed during the heating process. Therefore, this is not living food. This is not gut healing food.

Finding real ferments

This is tricky. You may need to sleuth to find properly fermented foods to purchase or you can take the easier route and make them yourself. Even innocent looking plain organic whole milk yogurt can have odd ingredients. I recommend that you always read food labels before purchasing.

Here's one example of what I found. Clover organic whole milk yogurt has organic pasteurized milk, organic pasteurized cream, pectin, organic corn starch, and live active cultures. Pectin and cornstarch? Yuck! Real yogurt should have whole milk and live culture—that's it. Flavored yogurts are even worse. Don't expect to find real fruit in them.

Commercially live fermented foods are likely to be available in the refrigerated section of your local health food store. Two reputable companies that ship real sauerkraut are listed on page page 133. The Weston A. Price Shopping Guide is another good reference for locating real fermented foods and real whole foods.

Defining the term "Properly Fermented"

Most of the literature and certainly many food scientists and biochemists agree that lactofermentation is an anaerobic process. Anaerobic means fermenting food in an environment without oxygen. Many books with fermentation recipes have you doing this in less than ideal circumstances. Many recommend using a mason jar that is tightly sealed. Hmm…close but not really….the grooves along the top of a mason jar lid allow for Grand Canyons of air compared to the size of the lactic acid bacteria trying to dominate the container of vegetables or whatever we are attempting to ferment. If oxygen can enter, then this also means that mold and undesirable yeast can enter, too. This is not good. The point of fermenting is to create healthy LAB bacteria to repopulate our gut flora and improve our overall health.

Aerobic ferments such as kombucha, vinegar and natto do need oxygen to ferment. Kombucha is covered in detail in the first section of Ferments.

Wild versus controlled ferments

My definition of wild versus controlled fermentation is as follows: **Controlled** ferments are made in Pickl-It jars or other anaerobic containers where airborne bacteria and yeasts cannot enter during the fermentation process. The cultures actively involved are either 1) present in fresh vegetables, 2) an added culture like kefir grains, 3) as a starter such as yogurt or the Caldwell starter or a combination (Caldwell and potatoes). All the fermentation recipes in the book are controlled except for kombucha. **Wild** ferments (aerobic) depend, to a degree, on the bacteria and yeast that is airborne in that particular environment. So it's more of a wild ferment since you cannot control it.

This distinction is important when fermenting foods as part of gut healing protocol such as the GAPs diet, Candida, or other health treatments. I hear regularly from many of my clients that the foods from the Pickl-It are the first ferments that they have been able to tolerate and actually enjoy without gastric distress. This is the benefit of a controlled anaerobic environment for people with less than ideal health conditions.

Pickl-It jars

I only endorse a closed-air system for lactofermentation (unless you are making kombucha or vinegar; these two products need oxygen to ferment). The Pickl-It jars are the device that I recommend if you want to make your own cultured foods. They are designed to optimize the proper conditions for successful fermentation. These jars are hermetically sealed and allow for the CO2 and extra fermentation gases that occur during fermentation to release through an airlock with a water barrier. So no exploding jars while maintaining the ideal environment for the LAB to quickly multiply. The materials used for the jars are carefully sourced to be free of environmental toxins. The owners of Pickl-It have chosen to use Italian glass both for the jars and "Dunk'R" (a weight used to keep vegetables submerged) and silicon food-grade grommets and Plug'R instead of the petroleum products that are commonly used by other producers.

The wide range of sizes also lends itself to easily fit your household's needs for various ferments. Whether you live alone or in a pack, like the Waltons, there is a size that is just right for your needs. The range of sizes is also convenient for making smaller batches of quick ferments such as dairy kefir, mayonnaise and salsas. I don't know many families who need to make a gallon of mayonnaise at a time. Another plus is that they are affordable. You could purchase several Pickl-It jars for the price of just one Harsch crock.

Weighing in on whey, starters and previous brines

Whey, vinegar and previous brines are not recommended (or needed) to kick start a new batch of ferments in the Pickl-It jar. These ingredients actually interfere with the lactofermentation process. Whey is a dairy culture, which is not useful or necessary for vegetable ferments. Whey actually interferes with the natural stages that LAB bacteria need to reach the correct pH and nutrient development as well as breakdown and consumer the antinutrients. End product LABs are different than initial LAB (Read **Lactofermentation Stages** on page 38).

So, why do most recipes in *Nourishing Traditions* and some other fermentation books include this as part of the recipe? Good question. Here's my opinion. If you are fermenting in a mason jar or other vessel where air is able to get in and out, then the whey would serve as an inoculant or vaccine for your ferment. Another negative of using jars that are not airtight is that the salt content has to be higher and the duration of the ferment is cut short to avoid spoilage and mold. But a shortened duration does not allow the ferment to complete all the stages of LAB fermentation.

There are a few exceptions to utilizing a starter. If you have:

- Not ideal sources of vegetables or vegetables grown in mineral depleted soil
- Frozen vegetables
- Potatoes or sweet potatoes and want to reduce acrylamide and starch/sugar

The only starter that I recommend is Caldwell broad spectrum starter. It is meticulously sourced from organic vegetables and not from a dairy source. I do not recommend Body Ecology (a narrow-spectrum starter base on dairy). See page 133 for sources.

Keys to successful fermenting

Darkness: Lactic acid bacteria and other enzymes thrive in darkness. All the recipes included in this book prefer darkness. Be considerate and give them privacy to multiple and do their jobs. You can tuck them away in a cupboard or closet or simply wrap a dish towel around the jar (leaving the airlock to stick out).

Temperature: Ferments are temperature sensitive. I have specified the appropriate temperature ranges with each recipe. Some ferments like warmer temperatures like dosa and kefir and most vegetables need lower ones. You will need to pay particular care when fermenting anything with cabbage. If your home temperatures are too cold for some ferments (like dosa and kefir) consider using a seedling heat pad or a dehydrator to assist you (see **Equipment** on page 131).

Salinity: The correct salt concentration is essential to successful fermenting. Salt is required by the lactic acid bacteria (LAB) to multiply and dominate the bad bacteria that can lead to spoilage. LAB are not able to out compete the bad bacteria if salinity is below the correct amount. Too much salt does not allow the LAB to thrive, and you end up with a salt cured product rather than a probiotic. A minimum 1% salt concentration is required for LAB to survive. Please see **Figuring Out Salt** on page 28 to easily calculate the grams of salt needed for brines.

Duration: The duration for a ferment to be complete and ready to eat is based on biochemistry. There are certain stages that occur during fermentation. I've included a summary of the steps involved (page 38), but you can read the complete details on the Pickl-It website. Just remember some foods are "slow foods" and are worth waiting for. Cabbage takes much longer than most other ferments in this book, but the payback in probiotics density and flavor are immeasurable.

How to use the Pickl-It

Detailed instructions are on the Pickl-It website, but here is my short version:

1. Always start with a completely dry, clean jar.

2. Fill the jar to its shoulder. Unless you are making a cabbage-based ferment, leave another inch available for the brine covering to come to the shoulder of the jar.

3. Close and seal jar. Check to make sure D-ring piece is attached as well as white gasket liner between the lid and jar.

4. Add airlock with water and top. Ferment at room temperature away from direct light. Use a towel to wrap sides if needed (leaving airlock out).

Ferment FAQs

Hey, isn't lactofermentation dairy stuff?

Not really. Lactofermentation is often confused as being dairy-based because of the prefix "lacto." This is not accurate. It does include dairy ferments, but the term itself refers to the bacteria that is created, lactobacillus or lactic acid bacteria (LAB). This is an important distinction because this allows individuals who are lactose or casein intolerant to still benefit from lactofermented foods.

Why use the airlock in the fridge? What do airlocks do?

The airlock "burps" the jar, so you don't have to. If you used the Plug'R too soon, you have to "burp" it—quickly pulling it out and reinserting it—at least once a day during the early, active stages. A healthy fermented food is a living fermented food; therefore, gas is always created, so it needs to escape the Pickl-It container.

Is there air or oxygen in the head space between the top of the brine and the lid of the Pickl-It container? Initially when you close the jar, yes. But as fermentation starts, layers of different gases are produced. They each have different molecular weights and functions. Some lock in flavor, while others color. When they accumulate beyond the capacity of the head space, they escape up and out the airlock.

Airlocks have been used for thousands of years. They are created and used for wine and beer-making, which must be created within an anaerobic stage. If wine wasn't created using anaerobic conditions, and oxygen was allowed in, the result would be vinegar.

How did traditional cultures ferment without the Pickl-It?

Fermentation pits were used for thousands of generations. A sealed porous crock was put into a wood or plant-lined pit, then covered with more plant material, then the entire pit was sealed with a cover. Gases created in the crock pushed oxygen out of the porous clay walls of the crock. Next, the lighter gases, as well as beneficial bacteria moved through the clay jar, filling up the airspace in the fermentation pit, inoculating all its surfaces. Eventually, the fermentation gases—all of which are heavier than oxygen—

pushed all the oxygen out of the chamber, creating an anaerobic chamber. Pickl-It is your modern day solution to not having a fermentation pit.

How long does fermented food usually last once I begin to use it?
All fermented foods have different life spans. Lactofermented salsas or chutneys are created and eaten within a few weeks. Lactofermented lemons need 30 days on the counter cure time and will easily last more than a year. The Pickl-It was designed for harvest-to-harvest preservation of fermented foods.

Will the brine last longer if the kraut is not in it?
The brine is the most essential part of a cabbage ferment. It is an extraction of the important probiotics and nutrients from the food. As long as the cabbage has carbohydrates remaining in its cells, in order to feed the lactic acid bacteria, your ferment is alive and well. Brine stored on its own will no longer have a food source and will decay over time.

How will I know if fermented food is bad? (e.g., smelly, moldy, etc.?)
If you made moldy, smelly, stinky, slimy batches of food with the Pickl-It, this may be what happened:

- No water in the airlock or you forgot to place the plastic cover on the airlock
- Washed the lid and gasket but didn't reinstall the white lid-gasket. Without this, it's not an airtight seal.
- Lost the D-ring that locks the bottom wire to the bottom jar. It's not possible to get anaerobic condition without this piece holding it tightly together.

What's the white stuff on my ferment? (This is rare)
This is rare, but it can happen. Yeast plays an important roll during lactofermentation. This yeast is called Kahm yeast, and it looks white, velvety, and powdery. Although harmless, Kahm yeast is something you **don't** want to overgrow since it affects the flavor of the ferment. Kahm yeast is typically caused by under salting or exposure to air. If your jars are clean, add enough salt so the ferment is sufficiently acid (primarily when it's started), and use airtight jars then it won't happen. If it does, you can safely skim it and add more brine (2% salinity). Kahm yeast is often cultivated for a yeast starter for beer, ale, or bread.

Can I ferment anything?
Not really. Some foods cannot be fermented or it simply doesn't make sense to try. Like guacamole, mashed avocados are already extremely digestible and are typically not an inflammatory or allergenic food. (That's why it's a good starter food for babies.) Also, it doesn't have much sugar or starch to feed a ferment. One online recipe that I am often questioned about has you mix all the ingredients with whey and let sit on the counter covered with plastic to "ferment" for seven hours. A layer of brown occurs on the top. Skim it or mix it back in, the recipe advises. I would disagree. This is oxidized food that is not good. It is not fermented. Canned food or food that has been fully cooked cannot be fermented either. This is no longer living and cannot be revived.

Ferments

Tips for Successful Fermenting

Keep your lactic acid bacteria happy by choosing:

- High-quality, pesticide-free ingredients (organic preferred)
- Antibiotic-free milk, as antibiotics will kill lactic-acid bacteria (grass-fed raw milk is best)
- Filtered water without fluoride or chlorine (both kill lactic-acid bacteria)
- Unrefined, high-mineral salt
- Cover Pickl-It to block UV light (do not cover the airlock)
- Salt is important. Follow the guideline and do not omit it.
- Follow the specifications for **duration** time for each ferment recipe
- Follow the specifications for **temperature** for each ferment recipe
- If temperatures are too cold in your home, try a seedling heat mat.
- Properly store your ferment for optimized LAB levels.
- Remember most ferments are condiments, so use small portion sizes, especially when first starting to add these to your diet.

Tips Specific to the Pickl-It

Keep your lactic acid bacteria happy by following all the tips in the box above. Then add these, too:

- Start with a dry, clean jar (unless you are making dairy kefir).
- Fill your jars with no more than 25% airspace at the top to start. I suggest to the shoulder of the jar, but the minimum is 3/4 full.
- Add water to the airlock and be sure to add the cover to the top!
- Make sure all the parts are working on the jar when closing. Make sure the D-ring is attached and the white gasket installed.
- Never have more than 50% airspace as you are using the ferment. Move it to a smaller jar to keep that airspace closer to 25%. Fermentation never stops and the LAB are sensitive to air. More airspace = less LAB
- If the airlock is no longer being used, be sure to use the Plug'R
- I recommend keeping a separate Pickl-It jar for dairy ferments. Milk proteins are difficult to completely remove from glass and may interfere with a vegetable ferment. Likewise, a jar used for fermenting garlic may not add a flavor that is pleasing to your dairy kefir.

Beverages

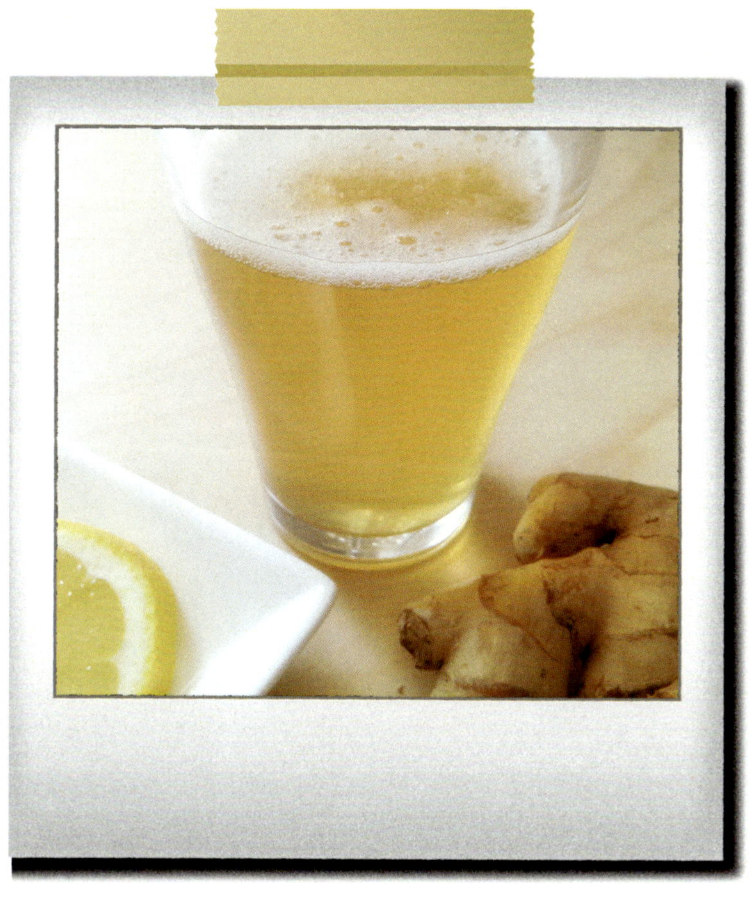

Kombucha

About Lactofermented Beverages

Lactofermented beverages have been made since Biblical times. They are fermented by lactic-acid forming bacteria, such as the probiotics present in our own gut and in cultured dairy products like buttermilk, yogurt and kefir. Most lactofermented beverages have a very low alcohol content, as the fermentation focuses on the formation of lactic acid as opposed to alcohol.

Perhaps the best known of lactofermented beverages is real root beer and ginger ale. Real apple cider is another example. Various forms of kvass are common in Eastern Europe and Russia.

Many of these beverages are healthful substitutes for syrupy-sweet sodas. While most of these are not particularly sweet, they are refreshing, invigorating, and healthful for our digestive systems.

Kombucha

Kombucha is a fermented tea made with a kombucha culture (aka mushroom, mother, scoby, etc.) tea prepared with sugar and some kombucha tea from a previous batch (aka starter tea). The mixture is allowed to ferment at room temperature for 5-30+ days. It can be consumed plain or with added flavoring. Kombucha contains a number of vitamins (particularly B-vitamins) and may have a number of health benefits.

There are a few things to remember about Kombucha. It is a forgiving culture, but it thrives in a clean environment and with temperatures above 65°F.

Kombucha creates glucuronic acid, which likes air. So the Pickl-It isn't a good choice since it is designed for anaerobic fermentation. Kombucha, on the other hand, **loves** oxygen. It needs oxygen to float across the top of its brine. A cloth napkin or loose-weave muslin is ideal as a cover.

Basic Kombucha

Makes 2 quarts

Kombucha can be divided into two stages—**Primary Fermentation** and **Second Fermentation**. The finished product after the first stage—when the tea is no longer sweet—is referred to as the Primary Fermentation. If you want to add flavor and fizz, add a Second Fermentation. Each stage is described after the initial recipe.

Primary Fermentation (at room temperature)

> **2 quarts water**
> **½ cup sugar (see kombucha FAQs on the next page)**
> **4 to 6 tea bags of black, green or white tea or a combo OR**
> **Lisa's Kombucha Tea—2 tablespoons**
> **½ cup or more of scoby/culture with starter tea**

1. Add sugar and water to a large pot. (Tip: heat half the water to be used and add the rest later to cool it quicker.) Bring to a boil. Turn off stove and add tea. Steep for at about 15 minutes.

2. Allow the liquid to cool to body/room temperature.

3. Add the sweet tea to the jar/container where the primary fermentation will take place.

4. Add the scoby to the tea (check to make sure tea is not too hot)—pour starter tea over the scoby.

5. Cover with cloth, lid to allow air circulation but keep fruit flies out. You can take the metal disk out of the 2-part mason jar lid and put the screw ring on over a piece of cloth napkin/paper towel. Keep the jar out of direct light.

Wait 7 days or more

After at least a week, taste the liquid. (This part is variable depending on temperature, scoby size and the quantity being made.) Kombucha ferments faster in warm weather. I find it takes at least 20 to 30 days in my house where it is quite cool—below 70°F during the summer and around 60°F or lower in the winter. I prefer a longer ferment so the sugar content left is minimal. The longer it ferments, the more of a tangy, sour flavor it will have. If you let it go too long, you get vinegar. You will know it is done when it does not taste like sweet tea.

When it's to your liking, you can take one of two paths:

1. Remove the scoby and store the plain kombucha (finishing fermented tea) in the fridge, making sure to reserve some of the finished fermented tea to cover the scoby for your next round of kombucha brewing; or

2. To flavor your kombucha and/or get more fizz. Proceed to the Secondary Fermentation.

Secondary Fermentation (at room temperature)

You need to first follow step one from the primary fermentation (set aside the scoby and a cup of the finished tea). Take some of the tea and add it to a bottle with a flip top lid or a glass jar with a screw lid– but more air will get in.

Add some flavor—examples are lemon juice, some chopped ginger and/or some raspberry purée. Flavor ideas: ginger, lemon juice, cranberry juice, pineapple juice— be creative! Add about 2 to 3 ounces for a liter of finished primary fermented tea. More options—add slices of watermelon, cucumber/celery, lemongrass, lemon/ cucumber, dried apricots, and so on.

Continue to ferment for several days—you may want to burp the jar or bottle every few days to make reduce the chance of any bottles exploding. This has never happened to me, but this is a risk. This second fermentation may take 4 to 5 days or longer in cooler weather. The jars/bottles should be kept out of direct light.

Cautiously open the flip top bottle in the sink **SLOWLY**. Test the tea for flavor and fizz. If it is to your liking, then move it to the fridge.

Backup scoby (store in fridge)

Tear or cut some part of the newer layer of your scoby, after your first two batches of kombucha, to serve as a backup. Just in case something goes wrong with your actively used scoby (your dog eats it or your toddler decides to play with it), you will have "extra." Be sure to add some new sweet tea every month or so to keep your culture fed. (The starter tea in the jar is great to add to your next batch of kombucha in the beginning.) Share extras with a newbie or compost, bury it with fruit trees, or give it to your chickens.

Kombucha FAQs

Starter Tea: This is the finished plain tea from the first fermentation or the tea you received with your scoby. Be sure to reserve a 1/2 cup of starter tea per 1/2 gallon water for your next batch. A good practice is to remove the scoby and place it in a clean bowl and cover it with your starter tea while you bottle your finished kombucha.

Water: Use filtered water that is free of chlorine and other toxins. Spring water and Reverse Osmosis water are good options.

Tea: Almost any type of actual tea, camelia sinensis, provides the nitrogen and nutrients kombucha requires. Along with sugar, it is the main fuel source for the culture/scoby. When you brew kombucha with herbal infusions, you may get a healthy fermented beverage. But over time, due to the lack of necessary nutrients, the culture will atrophy and eventually die.

I suggest using loose leaf, bulk, organic, fair trade (if possible). Loose leaf & bulk means less packaging (more green) and less costly. Organic fair trade is pesticide free (tea is often sprayed), and a fair wage is paid to those growing it.

Teas to avoid: Flavored teas such as Chai , Red Zinger or Earl Gray are often flavored with essential oils that may damage the culture.

Herbal infusions: These do not contain camellia sinensis. Some herbal infusions have volatile oils, which hinder the culture's growth and kill the lactic acid bacteria. I have not found that smoked teas make very tasty kombucha (but you might).

Over-fermented kombucha? A great replacement for vinegar, which you can use in almost any recipe. Good examples are dressings, marinades, and dips.

What the heck does SCOBY even mean? This is an acronym for **S**ymbiotic **C**ulture of **B**acteria and **Y**east, which is what the culture actually is.

Sweeteners:

- **Sugar:** The sugar isn't for you, it's for the culture (scoby). Sugar is the easiest food for the culture to ferment. I use organic, evaporated cane juice to avoid harmful chemicals from the bleaching process. Plain white sugar also works.

- **Molasses** is high in iron and is a by-product of sugar cane processing. It contains more iron, calcium, potassium and magnesium than table sugar. It may take the scoby a bit longer to break down the components of molasses before it gets to the sucrose. It can be substituted for sugar in a 1:1 ratio.

- **Honey** is antibacterial in nature and can harm the culture. You can use honey if it's **not** raw. Use 7/8 of a cup of honey for every 1 cup of sugar.

- **Stevia & Xylitol:** These are plant-based sugars and are not fermentable.

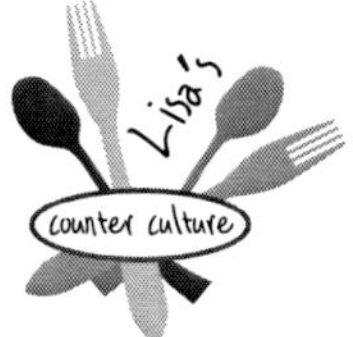

Beet Kvass

My first encounter with "beet kvass" was not that positive. I am not a fan of beets… they are okay when juiced with greens—but in my opinion, that's it. Yet when I began reading the books *Nourishing Traditions* and *Wild Fermentation*, I began to reconsider if only for the health benefits. I tasted a sample at a local farmer's market, and it wasn't awful. It was okay…but not good enough to buy. Later, I chatted with a friend who claimed that beet kvass can be really good if made correctly.

So like many recipes for fermentation, there was a lot of ambiguity on how to ferment the juice. And many of the recipes called for vague quantities of ingredients and differing lengths of fermenting time. I started trolling my collection of recipes at home and online and gathered some ideas on what to try. After a few failed batches, (mostly since I was not using an anaerobic Pickl-It), I made a batch that was actually quite tasty.

My children will immediately come to the kitchen if I yell out "beet kvass." They just love this stuff. They even like the fermented beets left over from making the tonic.

A good recipe can make all the difference. Be sure to read my recipe fully before you start. This will ensure that your first batch comes out great.

But before I share the secret to delicious beet kvass, let's talk about why you should consider drinking it. Fermenting beets greatly reduces the sugar content, so you are left with a very low sugar/carbohydrate and tangy beverage. Since it is lactofermented (dairy-free), it is full of lactobacillus and other beneficial bacteria and yeast (probiotics). During fermentation, the cultures are metabolizing the sugars in the beet cubes, converting them to lactic acid and CO_2, releasing the vital nutrients into the liquid. Beet roots can grow as far down as 10 feet into the soil, picking up trace minerals that have virtually vanished from the top layers due to repeated cultivation.

Like many fermented foods, beet kvass can improve digestion, restore the proper balance of bacteria in the gut, and add rich enzymes to make digesting easier and more effective. According to Sally Fallon (2000),

> *Folk medicine values beets and beet kvass for their liver cleansing properties and beet kvass is widely used in cancer therapy in Europe. Anecdotal reports indicate that beet kvass is an excellent therapy for chronic fatigue, chemical sensitivities, allergies and digestive problems.*

These nutrients include important trace minerals like calcium, magnesium, phosphorus, potassium, and sodium, and small amounts of iron, zinc, copper, manganese, and selenium. Beet kvass is a natural source of C and folic acid, vitamins B1, B2, B3, and vitamin A in the form of beta-carotene. It is also a good source of silica, which helps the body utilize calcium for healthy bones, skin, hair, and nails. The rich purplish reddish pigment of beetroot comes from betacyanin, which is a pigment that helps to prevent colon cancer.

Beet kvass may have originated in Ukraine, but is also enjoyed throughout Russian and Eastern Europe. I recommend drinking it in relatively small amounts, especially if you are new to fermented foods. It is considered a tonic drink, and if your system is out of balance, you may experience "die off." Some symptoms may include fatigue, digestive upset, low-grade fever, or dizziness/headache. So start smalland improve your gut flora balance slowly.

You may be able to find a local vendor selling beet kvass, but typically, it won't be properly fermented in a closed-air system or for long enough. If it is not fermented anaerobically, the chance of having a large population of good bacteria is significantly decreased while allowing undesirable yeast and bacteria to also take a spot. Are you ready to try making some of your own?

What is Die Off?

Unless you've been eating real food and avoiding all processed foods for a long time, chances are there is some kind of unbalance in your system even if you feel great. So it isn't surprising that our bodies will go through some change when we start ingesting beneficial bacteria. What happens is the balance is changed and the good bacteria start doing their job of balancing out the other flora in your gut. These cells die and release toxins. It sounds scary, but it isn't. This is where die off comes in. If you ingest a lot of beneficial bacteria, these other bacteria die quickly in large numbers and produce toxins faster than your body can clear them out. This is what causes the symptoms of die off. Don't be afraid of die off—you are leading your body back to better health.

Beet Kvass with Ginger/Cayenne

Pickl-It (I recommend the 1.5 Liter or 2-Liter jar to start) and a flip top bottle

Organic beets (peeled and chopped into 2 to 3 inch cubes)
Salt (2% brine or 20 grams salt for 1 liter water)
Ginger (peeled and sliced into 1 inch pieces)
Filtered water
1/8 teaspoon or less cayenne (optional, added after primary fermentation)

Important tips

- Fresh beets should be large and detached from greens for at least a week to concentrate the sugars.
- Try to choose beets that are at least the size of your fist.
- Make sure the beets are not cut too small or they will ferment too quickly.
- Vary the color and flavor of the final kvass by choosing different varieties of beets. Golden beets result in a beautiful orange tonic, Chioggia or striped pink/white results in a light pink tonic, and the traditional purple beets results in a deep wine colored tonic. The Chiogga and the golden beets are milder in flavor or less "beety."

Primary Fermentation

The key is to use 1/2 beet volume to 1/2 brine.

1. Place clean, peeled chopped beets into Pickl-It so that it is 1/2 of the volume.

2. Add a few 1 inch chunks of peeled ginger.

3. Make a 1.5 to 2% brine (I use 2% but 1.5% okay). Dissolve salt completely.

4. Fill brine to the shoulder of the jar. Add airlock with water. Ferment away from direct light at room temperature.

5. Ferment in a warm place (mid 70°F to low 80°F) for 7 to 9 days. You may see bubbles forming on the top. This indicates active cultures are thriving. Taste after several days. Mine usually takes at least 8 days, maybe longer in cooler weather.

6. It should not taste like salty water.
   Salty tasting—keep going with the primary fermentation.
   Not salty tasting—than proceed to the second fermentation or drink as is. I prefer the deep rich flavor that comes with the second ferment.

Secondary Fermentation (for fizz and depth)

Strain the beets and/or ginger and add the juice to a flip-top glass bottle.

Optional: Add less than 1/8 teaspoon cayenne or another flavor listed below, seal and let it ferment for a several more days at room temperature—even weeks. If it tastes good, then go ahead and move it into the fridge—it gets better over time. It will become richer, deeper in flavor, and perhaps fizzier. Some of my best kvass is several months old! I prefer to drink it cold.

More flavors: Try adding other herbs such as rosemary, turmeric, or even lavender during the second fermentation. Feel free to experiment!

Beet kvass FAQs

White yeast layer? If you see a thin white film on the top of the kvass—this is likely a harmless yeast called Kahm yeast—you can leave it or skim it. You may want to add a teaspoon of sugar to your next batch if this becomes an issue or try filling your jar with more beets, thus providing more sugar to feed the lactic acid bacteria.

Bubbles or foam on top? If you see bubbles on the top of the kvass while it is fermenting, this is nothing to worry about. This shows an active fermentation.

Can I eat the beets? The beets that are strained from the primary fermentation are now fermented or pickled. You may find them tasty. If so, save them in a light salt brine. Usually, I find that an additional few days in a 2% brine is needed. My kids love them, but I don't care for them—see what you think.

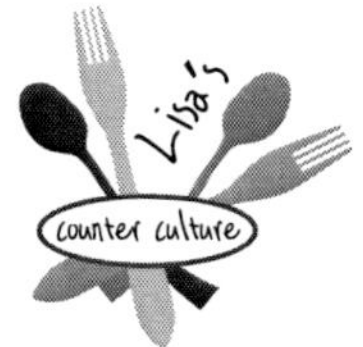

Water Kefir & Ginger Ale

Water kefir is made from water, sugar and water kefir grains. The culture is often referred to as a "grain" due to its crystal-like appearance. But it is not at all related to grains. It contains different strains of bacteria than kefir. It makes a nutritious, fizzy drink alternative to soda. The bacteria cultures in the kefir culture convert sugar to lactobacillus, which results in a lower sugar content and a tangy, fizzy flavor. However, sugar levels can vary, so use caution if you are diabetic or insulin resistant. Water kefir also contains B vitamins and can aid in digestion.

Water kefir is similar to milk kefir in that it is a probiotic-rich beverage, but water kefir is dairy-free, making it a great choice for people with dairy sensitivities. Water kefir is also a lighter beverage and can be flavored any number of ways, making it easier to drink larger quantities.

The different types of kefir have different benefits and drawbacks. Milk kefir is an excellent protein and calcium source, but contains some lactose, depending on how long you culture it. Water kefir does have a higher sugar content, but has many of the same vitamins and no lactose. Each type has different strains of beneficial bacteria, and they are easy to make at home, so try both!

Ginger ale or ginger beer uses culture or "bug" with ginger, sugar and water. This is what I call a "fun ferment" with not much punch in terms of nutrients and probiotics as compared to beet kvass or dairy kefir. Still, it's a worthwhile beverage with the healing properties of ginger and a probiotic component, too. Lactofermented ginger ale is helpful for soothing tummy aches, nausea, and menstrual cramps in addition to being refreshing and delicious.

Water Kefir Base

Adapted from *Eat Fat, Lose Fat* by Mary Enig and Sally Fallon

Kefir can be divided into two stages: a **Primary Fermentation** and a **Second Fermentation**. The finished product after the first stage—when the liquid has fermented for 12 to 24 hours—is referred to as the Primary Fermentation. If you want to add flavor and/or fizz, then add a Second Fermentation. Each stage is described after the initial recipe.

I recommend keeping your kefir grains "pure,"meaning that nothing is added to the primary fermentation, except for sugar water. Wait until you have enough extra grains to try experimenting with fermenting with juice, coconut water or other flavors during the **Primary Fermentation**. Details on why this is better is covered in the General FAQs following the recipes.

Primary Fermentation (at room temperature)

2-Liter Pickl-It

> **2 quarts filtered water**
> **1/2 cup sugar**
> **Water kefir grains (not a real grain, just looks like one)**

1. Add 1/2 cup sugar to 2 quarts of filtered spring water. Dissolve sugar. You may need to warm the water to completely dissolve the sugar.

2. Add sugar liquid to a 2-Liter Pickl-It jar with 3/4 cup water kefir grains and stir.

3. Close and add airlock with water. Cover with towel or ferment in cupboard.

4. Leave at room temperature for 12 to 48 hours.

5. Strain/remove (do not rinse) the grains and reserve the remaining kefir water for the second fermentation, or you can drink it as this stage if desired.

6. Add the grains to a new sugar water mixture and restart process at step 1.

Second Fermentation (at room temperature)

The **Second Fermentation** is for fizz and/or flavor. You can drink water kefir before this step if desired. After completing this second fermentation (when your desired flavor and fizz is reached), the kefir should be moved to the fridge for consumption and/or storage. Otherwise, it will continue to ferment at room temperature and may become too sour/alcoholic to drink.

Fermented Lemonade

1. Add the strained water kefir from the primary fermentation to a flip-top glass bottle or other bottle that you can seal tight.

2. Add 1 cup fresh lemon juice and cap. Ferment for 24 to 48 hours. Cautiously and slowly release the top in the sink to see if desired carbonation/flavor as been reached. Store in fridge when completed.

Other Favorites

- Reduce lemon juice to 1/2 cup and add 1/2 cup pineapple juice
- Add ginger slices to lemon juice
- ¼ cup fresh berry juice/pomegranate juice
- Add dried fruit such as apricots or plums.

Herbal Infusion Water Kefir: Mix one part finished water kefir (grains removed) with one part herbal infusion (e.g. Nettle Leaf, Red Raspberry Leaf, etc.). Herbal infusions can be made by combining a handful of fresh or dried herbs with one quart boiling water. Allow the herb and water mixture to sit for 6+ hours. Be sure the herbal infusion is completely cooled prior to mixing it with the finished water kefir.

Cream Soda Water Kefir: Make water kefir and remove the kefir grains. Add 2-3 teaspoons of high-quality vanilla extract per quart of water kefir. See *Eat Fat, Lose Fat* by Mary Enig and Sally Fallon for more flavoring ideas.

Water kefir FAQs

Can I flavor water kefir while it's brewing? Yes, technically you can add fruit (fresh or dried) to the sugar water at the same time you add the grains. I do not recommend this. Not all fruit is compatible with kefir grains and over time, this can damage the grains.

Can I use juice to make water kefir? Yes, straight fruit juice (organic is best) can be used to make water kefir. I strongly recommend getting your kefir grains established using sugar water (for at least a few batches) prior to using juice. It's good practice to keep separate sets of kefir grains for culturing juice and culturing sugar-water. Juice strains the integrity of the kefir grains (it helps to culture them in sugar water every few batches). I've found that using water kefir grains in juice and then sugar water doesn't taste good.

Can I use coconut water instead of sugar water? Yes, but follow the recommendations for the use of juice in the prior question.

What amount of kefir grains do I need to make water kefir? Three tablespoons of kefir grains will culture 2 to 3 quarts of water kefir every 24 to 48 hours

Where do I store my finished water kefir? Once the culturing process is complete and the grains have been removed, the water kefir should be moved to the fridge.

Can I use honey to make water kefir? Yes, but honey is antibacterial in nature and the water kefir grains are a mixture of bacteria in yeast. Therefore, honey is very hard on water kefir grains and will cause them to weaken (and eventually die). If you really want to use honey, plan on replacing your grains occasionally or try honey that is **not** raw.

Ginger Beer (Ale) "Soda"

Adapted from *Wild Fermentation*.
1 Liter Pickl-It for Part 1. Makes one gallon.

This is similar to a sourdough starter in that a "bug" is made and then added to the final ingredients to finish the recipe. Be sure to read through the entire recipe.

> **Large pot to hold at least one gallon easily**
> **Several flip-top bottles**
> **Rubber band, paper towel or coffee filter**
> **Fresh ginger root**
> **Sugar**
> **Filtered or spring water**
> **Strainer/fine mesh colander**

Part 1: Start Ginger Bug

This is going to be your starter or "bug," which you can use again and again. The ginger bug prefers temperatures above 75°F.

1. Chop 2 tablespoons of fresh ginger, cleaned but not peeled.

2. Add the chopped ginger to a 1-Liter Pickl-It.

3. Add I cup water. Do not use tap water! Chlorine kills all the good bacteria needed to make this work.

4. Add 1 teaspoon of organic cane sugar, stir vigorously. Close and add airlock with water. Cover with towel or ferment in cupboard at room temperature for 24 hours.

5. Every day, for the next 6 to 7 days, add another 1 teaspoon of organic cane sugar and a teaspoon of chopped ginger. Be sure to stir well each time. By the end of the week, the water will have become somewhat cloudy and you should see little bubbles. Now you have a live bacteria starter.

Part 2: Make the Base

1. Into a large pot, add 6 to 7 ounces of grated fresh ginger (I use the shred attachment for the food processor) to 3.75 quarts of water.

2. Add 1.5 cups of organic sugar.

3. Reduce heat and let boil gently for 20 to 30 minutes.

4. Let mixture cool. This is important: do not add the bug when the base is too hot or it will kill the good bacteria culture.

5. After cooling, add the juice of two lemons and stir.

6. Add most of the starter bug/water from the **Part 1**, reserving a few tablespoons of the bug to be reused for your next starter.

7. Mix the bug with the base, then strain the ginger pieces out through a fine-mesh strainer into a larger bowl or pot (minimum 1 gallon capacity).

8. Using a funnel, bottle the ginger beer into airtight bottles and leave in a dark place to ferment and get fizzy. Check in 5 to 6 days or sooner if room temperature is above 75°F.

9. Use extreme caution when checking your bottle. Open slowly in the sink. Ginger beer often gets quite active and can shoot out all over if the CO2 is not released slowly and carefully.

10. When fizzy, move to the fridge; otherwise, leave out at room temperature for a few more days.

Vegetables

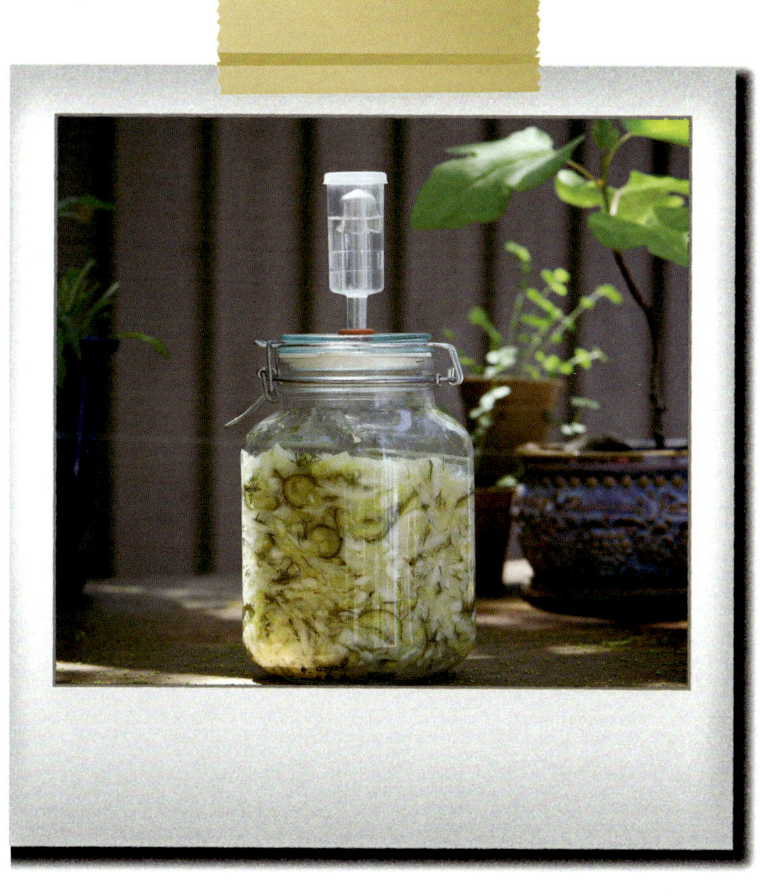

Figuring Out Salt

This is one topic that drives me crazy about fermentation recipes that I read from other sources. Salt is an important factor in fermenting! This is not added just for flavor. Salt has a specific function. If you have not read the **Required Reading for the Ferment Section** on page 3, then go back and read that part first for best results. Really, make sure you read this part.

The amount of salt brine needed is a ratio of salt dissolved into water and it is referred to as salinity. The only way to guarantee you are using the correct amount of salt is to use a gram-scale (see Equipment on page 131). Seriously, you need to weigh your salt. Salt varies widely due to its grind, density and moisture content. Think about it; this makes sense. A teaspoon of a dry fine grind salt will have a different weight than a moister, coarser salt.

I highly recommend using super fine Himalayan salt. (I covered why in the Introduction.) A big benefit to super fine grind salt is that it dissolves almost instantly, saving you the step of having to heat water to dissolve coarser grinds of salt and then waiting for the mixture to cool before you can add it to vegetables without cooking them.

Tip: 19 grams of salt dissolved in 1 quart of water results in a 2% brine.

Almost all vegetables require a 2% brine when using the Pickl-It system. Cucumbers are an exception with 3.5%.

- 2% Salinity: Green beans, carrots, broccoli, cauliflower, pearl onions, asparagus, green/red peppers de-seeded, parsnip, kohlrabi, zucchini, radish, mushroom
- 3.5% Salinity: Pickling cucumbers
- 10% Salinity: Brine-curing meat, feta-cheese, pepper-mashes, curing green olives, fish sauce.

I advise waiting until you are an experienced fermenter before tackling the 10% salinity ferments.

Handy brine table from the Pickl-It website

Water is measured in metric and salt is in grams.
Example: To create 2-liters of brine at 3.5% salinity, add 70 grams of salt.

	1-Liter	1.5 Liter	2 Liter	3-Liter	4-Liter	5-Liter
2%	20	30	40	60	80	100
3.5%	35	53	70	105	140	175
5%	50	75	100	150	200	250
10%	100	150	200	300	400	500

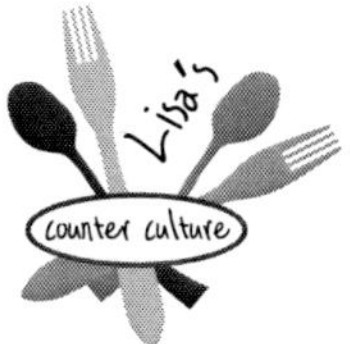

Condiments

Before modern canning, most of our American forbearers understood the process of lactofermentation. They had crocks of real sauerkraut, lactofermented cucumber pickles and other staples such as beets, onions or garlic stored during winter in the root cellar.

Many countries with longer histories than ours also traditionally fermented vegetables with salt, water and spices—knowing that this process would prevent the rotting of these vital nutrient-dense foods. Kimchi from Korea and cortido from Latin America are two examples.

When we lost touch with this preservation technique, we also lost touch with the health benefits that came with them. Sally Fallon is a devoted advocate of lactofermentation in her book *Nourishing Traditions*, and for good reason:

> *The proliferation of lactobacilli in fermented vegetables enhances their digestibility and increases vitamin levels. These beneficial organisms produce numerous helpful enzymes as well as antibiotic and anti carcinogenic substances. Their main by-product, lactic acid, not only keeps vegetables and fruits in a state of perfect preservation but also promotes the growth of healthy flora throughout the intestine.*

Lactofermentation is fairly simple, frugal and makes the most of your hard-earned real food. Lactic acid bacteria thrives in darkness so take care to shade your ferments.

I love condiments because they are so easy to incorporate with almost any meal. And they are kid-friendly, too. Almost any meal is improved by the addition of a delicious condiment—whether it is mayonnaise, salsa, chutney, dressings or dips. All these are probiotic-rich and great for digestion.

Tip: Wear gloves when cutting spicy peppers to avoid getting skin irritations from the chili oil. Wash your hands thoroughly after removing gloves as well. I learned this the hard way.

Lactofermented Mayonnaise

3/4 Liter Pickl-It

It is important that all ingredients are at room temperature. This mayonnaise is one of my favorite condiments since it can be the base for so much. Add it to salad dressings; add some to fresh shrimp or hardboiled eggs for a salad. Serve it with fish, chicken and burgers. Experiment to find your favorites. As long as you don't heat it, the cultures/probiotics are retained.

> **1 to 2 large organic egg yolks (no whites)**
> **1/2 teaspoon salt (2 grams superfine grind), more to taste**
> **1 tablespoon filtered water**
> **1.5 tablespoons lemon juice (add more to taste at end)**
> **1 cup olive oil (choose light and non-peppery)**
> **Options: pinch of mustard powder, pepper, and/or garlic**

1. Combine yolks, salt, water and lemon juice into processor. Blend for 30 to 45 seconds.

2. Add the oil slowly while processor is on. It helps to measure out your oil into a cup that pours well in a wire-thin stream.

3. When the emulsion becomes creamy, increase the speed with which you add the oil in a thin stream.

4. When all the oil is incorporated, add remaining lemon juice to taste. If the mayonnaise is too thick, add some filtered water. Taste and adjust seasonings if needed.

5. Add to Pickl-It and close the lid. Add airlock with water and ferment at room temperature for 3 to 4 hours in ¾ Liter Pickl-It with airlock away from direct light. Move to fridge.

Choosing the right olive oil: A less assertive olive oil makes a mayonnaise that tastes familiar. I discovered that low polyphenols usually translates into less "olive-oily" tasting olive oil. An olive oil with a more mild taste and with a more mild after bite generally gives the best results. In the bay area, Sigona's offers several low-polyphenol options, and you can taste before you buy. See Food Resources on page 133.

Tip: If the mayonnaise breaks or doesn't emulsify, don't despair. Reserve the blended ingredients into a cup. Add another yolk to the mixer/processor and try again.

Catchy Ketchup

1 Liter Pickl-It or Fido jar

Wait until you try this ketchup! You may never go back to store-bought. My kids insist on taking some with us when we go out for burgers. This is a more traditional and healthier version of commercial ketchup, but it's an acetic acid ferment rather than a LAB.

Note: This is not a lactoferment. Unless you dehydrate tomatoes to preserve the enzymes and bacteria needed for LAB fermentation and then make a paste, you will not be making a LAB cultured ketchup.

> **18 ounces unsalted tomato paste**
> **¾ cup water**
> **2 ounces Red Boat fish sauce (optional, but really makes it taste great)**
> **4 tablespoons apple cider vinegar**
> **1/4 teaspoon mustard powder (or prepared Dijon mustard)**
> **1/4 teaspoon cinnamon**
> **1/8 teaspoon cloves**
> **1/8 teaspoon allspice**
> **1/8 teaspoon cayenne**
> **1/2 teaspoon salt (reduce/omit if using fish sauce)**
> **1 to 2 cloves minced garlic or 1/8 teaspoon powder (or fermented garlic)**
> **1/4-1/3 cup raw honey or maple syrup**

1. In a medium sized bowl or food processor, whisk together all ingredients. Taste and adjust seasonings if needed. If too thick, thin with water or apple cider vinegar. This will thicken in the fridge.

2. Pour ketchup into the Pickl-It and close the lid with the Plug'R or use a Fido jar. Transfer to the fridge.

To make this a lactofermented ketchup: Use the Pickl-It jar with the following changes to the recipe. Make a paste using dehydrated tomatoes with filtered water for 18 ounces total. Leave out the vinegar and replace with lemon juice if desired. Use unrefined sugar, cooked honey or maple syrup to sweeten. Add all ingredients to the Pickl-It and close the lid. Add airlock with water and ferment at room temperature for 12 to 48 hours.

Salsa

Courtesy of Kathleen Mills, Pickl-It. Slightly modified.

Any salsa recipe can be fermented. Try mango, mango-peach, strawberry, or apricot. Experiment and discover new favorites. Here's how to convert your recipe for the Pickl-It.

1. **Leave out the vinegar and/or whey.**
2. **Add lemon or lime juice.**
3. **For every cup of fruit, add some or all of these items:**
   1/3 cup cilantro chopped
   1/3 cup onions chopped
   2 tablespoons lemon or lime juice
   5 grams salt
   1/8 teaspoon cumin

1. Mix ingredients in a bowl or process in food processer for finer texture.

2. Add mixture to Pickl-It and use a spoon to make sure all the chopped fruit pieces are below the liquid. Remove air pockets by stirring.

3. Ferment at room temperature (if below 74°F) for 5 to 14 hours with the airlock. Move to fridge. Ferment away from direct light. If warmer than 74°F, then ferment in fridge with airlock for 24 hours.

Watermelon Salsa

1-Liter Pickl-It

24 ounces diced watermelon
1/3 cup chopped cilantro
1 small red onion chopped
2 sprigs each mint and basil chopped
4 tablespoons lemon juice (or lime)
5 grams salt
1/8 teaspoon cumin
Teeny bit of chopped jalapeño (optional)

1. Mix ingredients in a bowl. I prefer to puree the lemon juice, salt and herbs together and a little of the watermelon to make enough juice to cover the ferment.

2. Add mixture to Pickl-It and use a spoon to make sure all the chopped fruit pieces are below the liquid. Remove air pockets by stirring.

3. Ferment at room temperature (if below 74°F) for 5 to 14 hours with the airlock. Move to fridge. Ferment away from direct light. If warmer than 74°F, then ferment in fridge with airlock for 24 hours.

Tomato Salsa

1-Liter Pickl-It or larger depending on size of tomatoes

A favorite! Vary the texture: you can make smoother by blending it or chunkier by hand-chopping the ingredients. Either way, it's delicious!

1/4 jalapeno chopped (optional—remove seeds or it will be spicy)
5 medium fresh organic tomatoes
Medium white or yellow onion chopped
2 garlic cloves minced
Several tablespoons fresh lemon or lime juice
5 grams salt
1/8 teaspoon dried oregano
½ bunch of cilantro chopped
Optional: add filtered water to thin

1. Add all ingredients to food processor or blender—pulse to desire consistency.

2. Add mixture to Pickl-It and use a spoon to make sure all the chopped fruit pieces are below the liquid. Remove air pockets by stirring.

3. Ferment at room temperature (if below 74°F) for 5 to 14 hours with the airlock. Move to fridge. Ferment away from direct light. If warmer than 74°F, then ferment in fridge with airlock for 24 hours.

Chutney, Converted

Courtesy of Kathleen Mills, Pickl-It. Adapted slightly.
1-Liter Pickl-It Jar

Basically, you take any chutney recipe, ignore the vinegar, and/or whey, reduce the sugar and make sure you use 1.5 teaspoons of salt per quart.

3 cups fruit (blueberries, pineapple, papaya, mango, plums, cherries, peaches, apples or nectarines)
1/3 cup minced onion (spring onions, Vidalia, yellow or shallot)
1/2 cup golden raisins or 1/3 dried currant
1/2 cup finely chopped nuts (pecan, macadamia, walnut, almond, cashew)
5 grams salt
1 tablespoon lemon juice
1 tablespoon grated ginger
1 teaspoon ground cinnamon
1/8 teaspoon ground allspice
½ or less red chili pepper, fresh or dried, no seeds, finely chopped
1/2-1 cup water

1. Mix all ingredients except for water; add to 1-Liter Pickl-It. Push mixture down with gentle pressure, trying to eliminate air pockets.

2. Add water, and again push ingredients down (or use a chopstick, poking down through brine, releasing trapped oxygen). The contents of the Pickl-It should be shoulder-high as the chutney will expand.

3. Place in Pickl-It jar, seal, add airlock and water.

4. Ferment at room temperature (if be;pw 74°F) for 5 to 14 hours with the airlock. Move to fridge. Ferment away from direct light. If warmer than 74°F, then ferment in fridge with airlock for 24 hours.

Note: For a sweeter version, add chopped raisins (to release sugars more quickly).

Fresh Mint Chutney

1-Liter Pickl-It Jar

> **1 bunch mint**
> **2 large, mature green onions or 1 small onion**
> **1 lime or lemon**
> **¼ to ½ cup filtered water**
> **½ to 1 teaspoon sugar**
> **5 grams salt**

1. Pluck mint leaves from the stems (discard stems). Peel onions and coarsely chop. Juice the lime or lemon.

2. Blend all the ingredients with 1 tablespoon lime or lemon juice, salt and ¼ cup water until well combined.

3. Taste and, if needed, adjust the amount of lime/lemon juice and salt.

4. Place in Pickl-It jar, seal, add airlock and water and ferment for 2 days, away from light, depending on temperature. Transfer to fridge.

Fresh Cilantro Mint Chutney

1-Liter Pickl-It Jar

> **1.5 cups firmly packed fresh cilantro**
> **½ cup firmly packed fresh mint leaves (or Thai or regular basil)**
> **1 Thai or red pepper flakes to taste**
> **2 inches ginger peeled and cut into chunks**
> **½ large red onion quartered**
> **2 cloves garlic peeled**
> **¼ cup freshly squeezed lime juice**
> **5 grams salt**

1. Blend the herbs, chili, ginger, onion and garlic until finely ground.

2. Add lime juice and salt. Blend.

3. You may need to add some filtered water to help the mixture blend.

4. Place in Pickl-It jar, seal, add airlock and water and ferment for 2 days, away from light, depending on temperature. Transfer to fridge.

Mango Chutney

Adapted from *Nourishing Traditions*
1-Liter Pickl-It

I like to blend the ginger, half the onion, jalapeno, mint, cilantro together with the remaining ingredients—leaving the mango pieces, red pepper, and other half of the onions chopped. This results in a smooth sauce with the contrasting crunch of red pepper, mango and onions.

3 cups ripe mango peeled and cubed
1 tablespoon freshly grated ginger
1 red pepper, seeded and cut into small pieces
1 small onion chopped
1 jalapeno chili, seeded and chopped (optional)
1/2 cup fresh mint leaves, chopped
1/2 bunch cilantro chopped
1/8 cup sugar
1/2 cup fresh lime juice
8 grams salt
1/2 cup water

1. Mix mango, ginger, peppers, onion, mint and cilantro in a large glass bowl.

2. Press down lightly with back of large spoon or other kitchen pounder.

3. Mix remaining ingredients well and pour over ingredients in the bowl.

4. Place in Pickl-It jar, seal, add airlock and water.

5. Ferment at room temperature (if below 74°F) for 5 to 14 hours with the airlock. Move to fridge. Ferment away from direct light. If warmer than 74°F, then ferment in fridge with airlock for 24 hours.

Variation: You can substitute papaya for the mango if desired.

Tip: Wear gloves when cutting spicy peppers to avoid getting skin irritations from the chili oil. Wash hands thoroughly after removing gloves. I've learned this one the hard way.

Cranberry Chutney

Here's a wonderful holiday recipe for traditionally fermented cranberry chutney. Best of all, you don't have to heat any of it! Great with almost anything—dosa, fish, chicken, etc.

1-Liter Pickl-It

12 ounces or 4 cups fresh cranberries (washed and toss bruised/mushy)
1/4 cup sugar
5 grams salt
3 to 4 small Satsuma or Murcott (tangy tangerine with seeds removed)
1 teaspoon cinnamon
1/8 teaspoon cloves
½ inch fresh ginger finely chopped
Juice from 2 lemons, or 1 lemon and 1 orange (orange makes it sweeter)

1. Peel and separate Satsuma or whatever mandarin/tangerine variety you are using. Be sure to remove seeds. Add to food processor or high-speed blender.

2. Add sugar, salt, cinnamon, cloves, ginger, lemon and/or orange juice. Blend.

3. Add cranberries. Pulse until cranberries are broken up,but you want to retain some texture, so don't over-process.

4. Place in Pickl-It jar, seal, add airlock and water.

5. Ferment at room temperature (if below 74°F) for 5 to 14 hours with the airlock. Move to fridge. Ferment away from direct light. If warmer than 74°F, then ferment in fridge with airlock for 24 hours.

Cherry Chutney

1-Liter Pickl-It
We like this chutney with goat cheese, fresh yogurt and buckwheat pancakes.

1.5 cups fresh cherries pitted
1/4 cup mint leaves minced
1/4 cup onion minced
5 grams salt
1 teaspoon fresh ginger minced
1 tablespoon sugar

1. Add all ingredients to a mixing bowl and combine well.

2. Ferment at room temperature (if below 74°F) for 5 to 14 hours with the airlock. Move to fridge. Ferment away from direct light. If warmer than 74°F, then ferment in fridge with airlock for 24 hours.

Lactofermentation Stages

The *Handbook of Functional Fermented Foods* (page 402) explains the step-by-step process of spontaneous lactofermentation with sauerkraut as an example. You can read this detailed description in the handbook or read this more easily digested (pun intended)version written by Pickl-It on their website.

I have condensed their post here, but you can read the full post on their site listed in the Fermenting FAQs section. Who knew this was happening in our ferments!

The steps that follow have to occur in the particular order presented because of biochemistry. This process is the same for all fermented foods whether they are vegetables, grains, dairy or fruits. It is important to note that this process shifts from aerobic to anaerobic—a critical step for the overall health and stability of the final brine and fermented food.

"Amazingly, anaerobic lactobacillus bacteria (LAB), the 'good guys', which are crucial and foundational to lactofermentation", are only available in **extremely** small numbers—only about 0.15 to 1.5% of the total bacterial population, primarily belonging to Leuconostoc mesenteroides ssp. mesenteroides at the beginning of the process."

- Step 1: Fermentation begins the moment the cabbage is filled into containers. Must be tightly packed so that aerobic bacteria (Pseudomonas, Flavobacterium, and Acinetobacter species—the microbes you do **not** want to have in your ferments) are deprived of oxygen, and are immediately diminished.

- Step 2: Shift in fermenting environment to anaerobic, with the salt and reduced pH working together, supporting the anaerobic lactic-acid bacteria (LAB), Leuconostoc mesenteroides. Depending on temperature, these first two stages are completed in 3 to 6 days. Lactic acid will have increased to approximately 1%.

- Step 3: Lactic acid bacteria shift to homofermentative LAB that dominate due to anaerobiosis, lowered pH and elevated levels of salt. The pH at this point is approximately 3.8 to 4.1 and results in a mild-flavored sauerkraut. This is when food processors in Europe typically unpack and pasteurize their kraut.

- Step 4: Only fresh, unpasteurized sauerkraut will undergo the final stage for full nutritional and flavor development. Stage 4 is typically takes at least 30 days with the proper fermentation conditions discussed earlier in this article. (Temperature, anaerobic, absence of light, etc.).

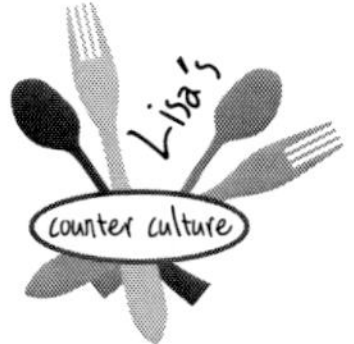

Sauerkraut and Kimchi

Cabbage ferments deserve its own section, as they are one of the more complex ferments in terms of biochemistry. All lactofermented foods go through three stages of fermentation. Cabbage-based ferments undergo a fourth stage of fermentation in non-commercial settings. Please read the previous page for details on these stages.

The fermentation process that I recommend uses traditional methods adapted to our modern world. We don't have fermentation pits. That's why I use the Pickl-It jars.

Numerous antinutrients are created during the first six weeks of cabbage fermentation. So eating it too soon is not a good idea. LAB bacteria require several vitamins, such as vitamin C, to power them through fermentation, which means early cabbage ferments are lacking in vitamin C if eaten too soon. Also, the chemistry that changes cabbage into sauerkraut takes weeks to rid the cabbage of its cabbage flavor. Sauerkraut should not taste like cabbage or too salty when properly fermented.

A common complaint with the mason-jar-whey or mason-jar-no-whey methods is that they are too salty. If whey isn't used in the mason jar, it is recommended by *Nourishing Traditions* to **increase** the salt. So the brine tastes salty if you left a mason jar ferment to cure for the Pickl-It recommended time of 8-12 weeks, the kraut is often loaded with oxygen-rich yeast (which are not probiotic, and feed Candida in the gut), and the kraut may well have turned color from green to brown, showing that it has been oxidized. This is obviously not desirable.

Properly fermented kraut, created in a true anaerobic environment, left to age for 8-12 weeks, does not taste like cabbage or taste salty. Vitamin C has been restored back into the ferment. This natural Vitamin C is needed to digest the sauerkraut.

Basic Sauerkraut

Modified slightly from the Pickl-It website.
1.5 Liter Pickl-It

2.5 pounds organic cabbage
30 grams salt
Pickle Kraut variation: Add thinly sliced cucumbers, three cloves crushed
garlic, and fresh chopped dill
Beet Kraut variation: Add 1 medium golden beet, peeled and grated
Classic Caraway variation: Add one teaspoon or more caraway seeds

1. Save two or three layers of outer leaves from the cabbage head. Grate/Chop the remainder.

2. As you add the cabbage to a large mixing bowl, sprinkle salt between the layers.

3. Leave for one hour or two.

4. By now the cabbage has started to weep. Squeeze cabbage with clean hands.

5. Add flavors or herbs if desired. Mix into cabbage.

6. Layer cabbage into the Pickl-It jar using a large spoon or a potato masher. Every few inches of layered cabbage/salt, push the air pockets out of the cabbage. Continue to build and push layers until the cabbage reaches the "shoulder" of the Pickl-It jar—a couple of inches below the "neck."

7. With an inch of brine covering the cabbage, add the cabbage leaves on top. Place the Dunk'R on top of the cabbage leaves (the leaves keep the shredded cabbage under the brine). Unlike other methods, you don't need to worry about oxygen-yeast or oxygen-mold forming inside the Pickl-It. The purpose of keeping the cabbage under the brine is so that the cabbage-sugars are removed by the LAB.

8. If there is not enough brine at the top yet, latch the cover on and place the Plug'R into the Pickl-It lid. Let the cabbage/salt sit in the Pickl-It for about 5 to 10 hours. Open the cover and press the cabbage down, pushing the brine out of the cabbage. The salt should have extracted enough brine to completely cover the cabbage. Ideally the brine is 1 inch above the cabbage.

9. Latch the Pickl-It lid. Place the large airlock into the lid-grommet. Add water to the airlock. Wrap a towel around the Pickl-It sides.

10. Place the entire Pickl-It in a dark corner of a 60 to 72°F room if possible. Refer to this table for specific recommendations on temperature and duration.

Temperature	Time	Location
Less than 72°F	3 to 10 days	Counter
Each degree above 72°F	Reduce the days by 2	Counter
73°F	Max 7 days	Counter
74°F	Max 5 days	Counter

11. Place in refrigerator with the airlock and allow the kraut to cure for a minimum of 10-12 weeks. This length of curing is traditional.

12. Alternatively, at temperatures 60°F and below, ferment/cure at room temperature for at least 6 weeks.

13. Wait to test the kraut around the 8th or 9th week. If it tastes salty or "cabbagey," it needs to cure for a few more weeks.

Cabbage ferment FAQs

Storage: Store in the Pick-It container. Anaerobic, traditional kraut, made in the Pickl-It has the potential for a year's storage in the refrigerator. As the kraut is reduced in the jar, and there's more head space created, it is important to move the kraut into a smaller Pickl-It to reduce the amount of head space.

Need a starter? If you are unsure when or where your cabbage was grown and the length of time it was stored, you may want to consider using Caldwell's Starter Culture. It will not hijack the natural, spontaneous fermentation, but instead, work in-sync as well as filling in any gaps of missing LAB. Also, the Caldwell's Starter Culture has a great recipe for adding more brine to the cabbage, which creates more juice.

Brine: Traditionally, the kraut brine or "juice" was valued as being the most important nutritional aspect of cabbage fermentation. The kraut fibers have always traditionally been added to soups, stews and cooked with food. Since the brine has extracted all the nutritional value from the cabbage, the kraut strands are actually just leftover fiber. So drink the brine and cook with the kraut for best nutrition.

I need kraut now! What can I eat while I wait for my kraut to finish?
Find a reputable source to hold you over during this waiting period. I know of two good companies that are fairly easy to access. Check Food Resources on page 133.

Kimchi My Way

Kimchi can be made with many variations so feel free to experiment. This is a very basic recipe but you can add or subtract ingredients to reflect the seasons or to include some of your other favorite vegetables. This can be as mild or spicy as you desire, simply adjust the red pepper powder or chili.

1.5 liter Pickl-It

1 to 2 heads Napa cabbage (about 2 pounds)
30 grams salt
1 or 2 onions chopped
1 to 2 bunches of spring onions chopped diagonal (use green parts only)
3 cloves of garlic
1 to 2 tablespoons red pepper powder (less for milder and more for spicy)
1 inch ginger root, peeled and chopped
1 ounce Red Boat fish sauce (optional)

1. Prepare a brine of 4 cups filtered water and 4 tablespoons sea salt. Mix to thoroughly dissolve salt.

2. Chop cabbage into 2-inch squares and place into the brine, covered with a plate to keep it submerged, for a few hours or overnight.

3. Add ginger, ginger, garlic, onion, and red pepper powder into food processor. Blend until it is a paste (aka spice paste).

4. Drain brine from cabbage, saving some brine.

5. Chop spring onion greens on a slant.

6. Mix cabbage and onion greens with spice paste. Wear gloves or use spoon. Pack tightly into the Pickl-It jar until liquid rises above the cabbage. If it is not submerged, add a little of reserved brine to cover.

7. Add Dunk'R and airlock with water. Store away from light.

8. Ferment at room temperature. Kimchi does best at about 65 degrees. So in warmer weather, ferment for a shorter time at room temperature and longer in the fridge.

9. Follow the instructions from the basic kraut recipe for temperature and duration specifics.

10. Place in refrigerator with the airlock and allow the kraut to cure for a minimum of 10-12 weeks. This length of curing is traditional.

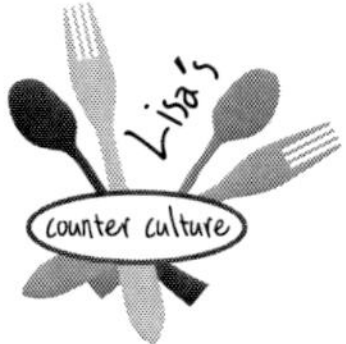

Vegetables

There are so many vegetables to ferment! Pickles are a favorite in our home—especially the half-sours. And the best thing about fermenting in the Pickl-It and then storing them in the same jar is that they keep for quite a while. We still have a few from our last harvest, and we are about to ferment this year's harvest. This is true harvest-harvest preservation without the loss of nutrients that you get when you can or heat process pickles.

I've included our top vegetable ferments (besides kraut and kimchi). But feel free to branch out and try new ones!

What to do with your leftover brine? Don't toss out this liquid gold! It's full of lively probiotic bacteria, and it tastes great, too! You can also use kimchi or kraut juice.

- Drink it up as a refreshing beverage
- Add it to fermented mayonnaise to make a dressing
- Add it to a salad dressing (cut back the vinegar to adjust to taste)
- Add it to egg or tuna salad—or one of my favorites—1/2 tuna and 1/2 egg salad
- Add a dash to dip for veggies
- Add to deviled eggs
- Add it to rice; it's especially good in sushi rice
- Add it to potato salad
- Add some zest to your soup—try adding to beet soup as a finishing touch—add it to slightly cooled soups or better yet cold summer soups
- Bloody Marys!
- Pickle juice popsicle—one of our favorites!
- Pickle juice is a great tenderizer for meat

Awesome Half-Sour Pickles

Adapted from *Nourishing Traditions* and *Wild Fermentation* and lots of practice.

Tips: Be sure to choose firm, fresh pickles that are of similar size. Snip the stems off close to the cucumber. Don't skimp on the salt—this will protect your pickles from becoming mushy.

Soak pickling cucumbers in a bowl of cool filtered water for 20 minutes, unless just harvested. This rehydrates the cucumbers so that they don't absorb the salt brine too quickly, and you end up with mushy pickles.

> **Pickling cucumbers to fit snugly into Pickl-It (Kirby variety works well)**
> **2 tablespoons fresh dill, snipped (flowering dill preferred)**
> **3.5% salinity brine (see Brine Table on page 28)**
> **Water**
> **1 to 2 grape leaves (optional: keeps cucumbers from going soft)**
> **Seasonings: peeled garlic cloves, peppercorns, thin slices fresh jalapeño, celery seeds, mustard seeds**

1. Wash fresh firm cucumbers well and be sure to snip off any stems. Don't scrub off natural beneficial yeast and bacteria.

2. Add garlic, dill, seasonings and grape leaves to the bottom of the jar

3. Place cucumbers into the jar so that they fit in snugly and are below the collar of the jar

4. Dissolve salt in water. Pour over cucumbers, adding more water if necessary to cover the cucumbers. The top of the liquid should be at least 1 inch below the top of the jar or to the collar of the jar.

5. Place Dunk'R on top to keep the cucumbers submerged. Cover and be sure the cucumbers are below the brine. Insert airlock and fill with filtered water.

6. Keep at room temperature for about 4 to 5 days before testing to see if the pickles are done. Be sure to keep a towel wrapped around the jar or place the jar out of direct light. You may need to keep for a few more days, depending on the ambient temperature. Transfer to the fridge for storage when they are done to your liking.

Note: Pickles will continue to ferment slowly in the fridge. So if you prefer a less sour pickle, than err on the side of caution by moving to cold storage a day or two early. Keep the brine when the pickles are done!

Dilly Beans or Carrots

1-Liter Pickl-It

1.5 pounds fresh firm snap beans washed and stem ends removed.
2 tablespoons fresh dill, snipped (flowering dill preferred)
20 grams salt (2% salinity)
1 pint water
1 to 2 grape leaves (to keep beans from going soft)
Seasonings: garlic, peppercorns, a few slices of fresh spicy pepper, celery seeds, mustard seeds.

1. Add garlic, dill, seasonings and grape leaves to the bottom of the jar

2. Pack beans into the jar so that they fit in snugly and are below the collar of the jar

3. Dissolve salt in water. Pour over beans, adding more water if necessary to cover the beans. The top of the liquid should be at least 1 inch below the top of the jar or to the collar of the jar.

4. Add the Dunk'R and make sure the beans are submerged.

5. Cover with lid and airlock with water added. Keep at room temperature for about 4 to 5 days before transferring to the fridge. Be sure to taste first and see if it needs a few more days on the counter. Keep out of direct light or cover the sides with a napkin and clothespin. Lactic acid thrives in darkness.

Note: When the green beans are gone, keep the brine, which is full of good bacteria. Drink up, add to salad dressings, mayonnaise, or dips.

Alternative: Try carrot sticks instead of green beans. No need for grape leaves with carrots or most other harder vegetables. This recipe also works well with cauliflower, romanesco, and mixed vegetables like carrots, cauliflower and broccoli.

Spiralized Daikon

This is a surprising delicious ferment. Daikon is like cabbage in that it will make its own brine. Adding salt over the shredded pieces will make it weep. Light squeezing and packing the jar will provide enough brine to submerge it. It's amazing how much brine it creates!

I use my Vegetable Spiral Slicer (see page 131)), which cuts the daikon into long thin spirals. You can also use a mandolin or a knife to thinly slice the daikon. The key is to get very thin pieces.

2-Liter Pickl-It

3 large organic daikon peeled
20 grams salt (2% salinity)
2 cloves garlic finely minced
1/8 teaspoon ground coriander

1.   Process peeled daikon through the spiral slicer and place into a large bowl

2.   Generously sprinkle super fine Himalayan salt on daikon

3.   Let it sit for 20 minutes. The daikon will release a lot of water/brine

4.   Massage/mix daikon to get the salt evenly distributed. If there is a lot of brine than add the garlic and coriander and mix it in. If there is not enough brine, then spend a few more minutes massaging the mixture. It will release more when you pack into the Pickl-It jar.

5.   This usually is enough to fill a 2-Liter jar when I make it, but you may need to adjust the jar size depending on the volume of your batch.

6.   Pack it tightly into the jar. Be sure to remove any air pockets. The brine should cover the top of the daikon by a 1/4 inch.

7.   Close lid and add the airlock with water. Leave at room temperature for 6 to 7 days, out of direct light. Transfer to the fridge with the airlock and let cure for at least two more weeks. It just gets better and better as it ages.

Dairy Ferments

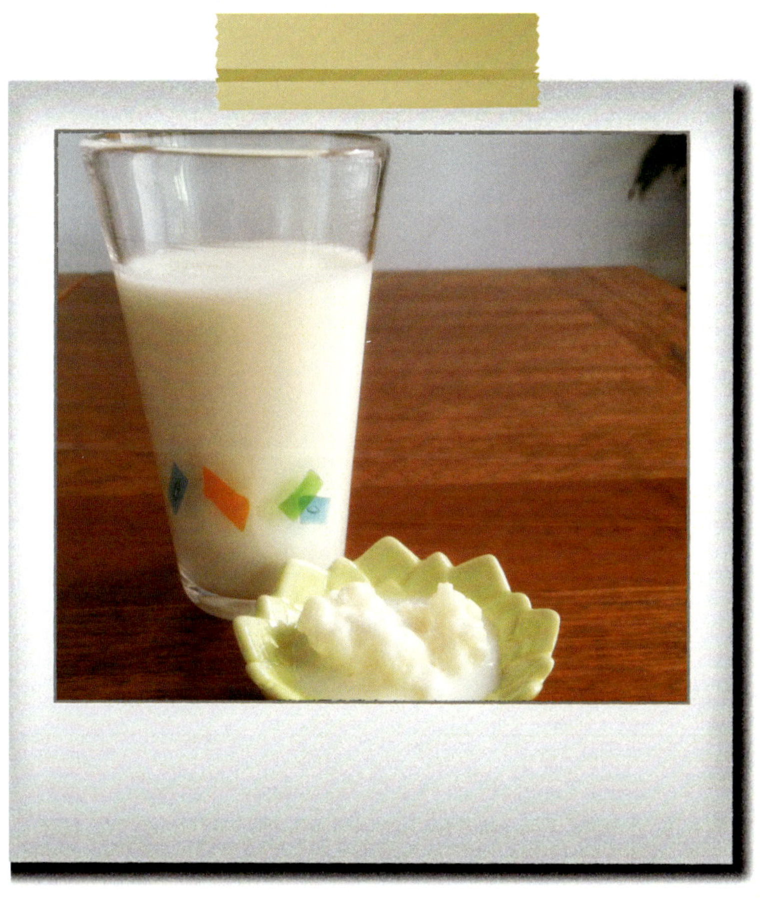

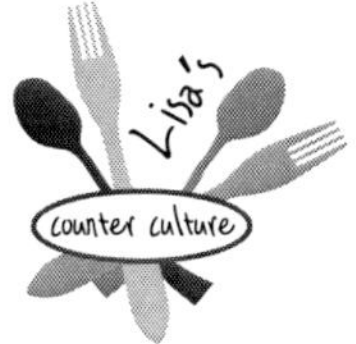

Kefir and Yogurt

Dairy Kefir

Did you know there are two types of kefir? Milk kefir is more commonly found than water kefir in the dairy department of many grocery stores. Both use a symbiotic culture of bacteria and yeast to ferment different bases (milk versus sugar water). The culture is often referred to as a "grain" due to its cottage curd or crystal-like appearance. But it is not at all related to grains.

Milk kefir is the traditional form of kefir, and it has been made for hundreds of years. It contains many of the benefits of milk, including high protein content, calcium and other minerals. Kefir is also a rich source of B vitamins, including folic acid. Milk kefir is usually low in lactose, and if you are lactose intolerant, you may be able to drink it. It also contains some dietary fiber. Milk kefir may upset your stomach at first if you aren't used to it, so it is recommended that you start with small amounts.

Making kefir is easy and much more affordable than buying it. You can use any type of milk, except ultra-pasteurized milk. This is a dead food that you cannot revive by fermenting it with a culture.

Choosing Milk

Milk quality is essential. Here's how I rank my choices. First is whole raw, then grassfed, then organic, then goat over cow, then pasteurized but **not** homogenized. What does this mean?

Raw is fresh whole milk produced without any other processing. No cream removed, no heat, just cooling and bottling.

Pasteurized milk is heated and held at a high temperature, resulting in the loss of valuable enzymes such as lactase (which is needed to break down lactose) and the beneficial bacteria that protects it from undesirable pathogens and other nutrients.

From the Weston A. Price Foundation website:

Not only does pasteurization kill the friendly bacteria, it also greatly diminishes the nutrient content of the milk. Pasteurized milk has up to a 66 percent loss of vitamins A, D and E. Vitamin C loss usually exceeds 50 percent. Heat affects water soluble vitamins and can make them 38 percent to 80 percent less effective. Vitamins B6 and B12 are completely destroyed during pasteurization. Pasteurization also destroys beneficial enzymes, antibodies and hormones. Pasteurization destroys lipase (an enzyme that breaks down fat), which impairs fat metabolism and the ability to properly absorb fat soluble vitamins A and D. (The dairy industry is aware of the diminished vitamin D content in commercial milk, so they fortify it with a form of this vitamin.)

We have all been led to believe that milk is a wonderful source of calcium, when in fact, pasteurization makes calcium and other minerals less available. Complete destruction of phosphatase is one method of testing to see if milk has been adequately pasteurized. Phosphatase is essential for the absorption of calcium.

Homogenized is a process that breaks up the fat globules and evenly distributes them throughout the milk so that they do not rise. This denatures the protein in the milk and makes it vulnerable to oxidation.

The most digestible milk commonly found in the U.S. is organic raw goat milk kefir. But you need to choose the option that works best for your situation. See page 133 for help finding real milk.

Dairy kefir FAQs

Rinsing: Do **not** rinse the grains between batches unless they stop making kefir effectively (which can sometimes be attributed to a build up of yeast on the grains). If it becomes necessary to rinse the grains, use milk! There is a protective barrier around these precious grains that can be greatly harmed with water rinsing.

To stir and shake? Up to you. This sometimes helps to see how far along it is.

Vacation or a break: Put the kefir grains in fresh milk, store in a Pickl-It with the airlock tucked in the back of the refrigerator. The cold will cause to culture to become somewhat dormant. Depending on the ratio of milk to grains in the jar, several weeks should be fine. Higher milk to grain ratio = longer storage.

Ferment cross contamination: This is not really an issue with closed air fermentation. However, I would keep kombucha (open air ferment) or sourdough (if it's not in a Pickl-It) away from the kefir, just to be on the safe side.

Curds and whey: Kefir may separate if it over-cultures. When this happens, I usually stir it a bit and then proceed. If it tastes too sour, try adding some fruit. To prevent future separation, reduce the length of time the kefir ferments and/or lower the temperature if too warm. Consider finding a cooler spot in your home.

Washing the Pickl-It jar: I have one (okay, really two jars, one for goat and one for cow) dedicated to only dairy kefir. I always use these two jars. I do not wash them between batches. Milk proteins are notoriously difficult to completely remove from most surfaces, glass included. Plus, I already have these great cultures coating the jar. So I simply strain the grains, reserve the completed kefir, add grains back to the jar with fresh milk and keep going. One less thing to wash! Of course, if something funky happens to your kefir (this has never happened to me) then wash and dry it fully.

Dairy Kefir

1-Liter Pickl-It

> **Milk**
> **Kefir grains**

1. Take a teaspoon of kefir grains (you can leave the milks stored with the grains) and place into the Pickl-It jar. You do **not** need to strain the grains out of the milk or rinse the grains.

2. Add milk to the shoulder of the jar.

3. Close the jar and add the airlock with water. Place the jar away from direct light.

4. Leave kefir at room temperature. When the kefir has thickened and tastes tangy to your liking, it is ready to strain out the grains and eat. Kefir prefers temperatures in the mid 70s°—and will ferment much faster in the 80's°. Be careful not to over ferment as it may separate into curds and whey.

5. Kefir generally takes 12 to 48 hours. The exact amount of time will vary depending on temperature and ratio of grains to milk. Cold retards the fermentation process, so kefir will form more slowly in a cold area (and can be all but stopped by placing the grains in milk in the refrigerator). Heat speeds the process, so kefir will form more quickly in a warm area and will be more likely to over culture. I recommend standard room temperature whenever possible. Allowing the kefir grains to remain in milk longer than 48 hours risks starving the kefir grains and potentially damaging them.

6. Strain the kefir grains from the milk, but do not overstrain and lose your grains through the strainer! Kefir is ready to drink or use in a recipe.

7. Place the grains in a new batch of milk and restart the process.

Favorite smoothies

Blend 1 pint of kefir with these variations:

- 1 banana and 1 teaspoon of raw cocoa powder
- 1 cucumber, generous pinch of salt
- Small handful of fresh berries
- Add some vanilla, pinch of cinnamon or pumpkin pie spice
- 1 to 2 tablespoons of almond butter
- Add lemon peel for a second ferment at room temperature (with grains removed)

Avocado Cilantro Kefir Dip

Makes 1 quart. (Soup and Dressing, Too)

I created this soothing recipe as a healthier version of a cool summer soup that I liked at local grocery. But I wanted a probiotic of these flavors. So this recipe soon became a favorite in our home. I often serve it in a small bowl as a snack, but the kids prefer to dip veggies in it, or you can thin it with more vinegar or filtered water for a great salad dressing. I've also served it along with grilled fish and as a soothing counterpoint to a spicy curry.

Handful fresh cilantro
2 small cucumbers peeled and seeded
1/2 avocado maybe more
1 pint milk kefir
Lemon juice (a few tablespoons)
Salt and white pepper to taste
Clove garlic minced
Pinch cayenne (optional)

1. Add cilantro to food processor and blend well.

2. Add garlic and cucumbers and blend some more. Scrape the sides down as needed. Add avocado. Blend more.

3. Add seasonings, lemon juice and kefir. Blend until smooth and creamy.

4. Taste and adjust seasonings as needed.

Note: This will thicken in the fridge. Best when consumed within 4 to 5 days, as it gets more sour with time.

Kefir Ice Cream

Makes 4 (small) servings

1/2 cup milk kefir
Two to three sliced frozen bananas
Teaspoon cocoa powder or chopped dark chocolate
Handful chopped dried cherries
¼ cup ice
Raw honey (optional)

1. Place ingredients in high-power blender or food processor with frozen banana and ice at the bottom.

2. Blend and serve soft or freeze for firmer texture. Add raw honey to sweeten as needed.

Kefir Pistachio Pesto

1 cup shelled unsalted roasted pistachios
½ cup fresh basil leaves and/or cilantro
1/4 cup chopped fresh flat leaf parsley
1/2 cup kefir
1/4 cup Parmesan cheese, preferably raw milk Parmesan
1/2 cup extra virgin olive oil
2 cloves garlic minced
2 tablespoons fresh lemon juice
1/2 teaspoon salt or to taste
White pepper to taste

1. In a food processor, process the pistachios, basil and parsley until fine.

2. Add kefir and the rest of the ingredients and process until pesto is well combined.

3. Taste and adjust the seasonings if needed.

4. Serve immediately or store in an airtight container in the refrigerator. Bring to room temperature before serving. Serve with cherry tomatoes, celery sticks, crudités or buckwheat crackers.

Kefir Leather

They are great for traveling. And if you dehydrate them at 135°F or below, the kefir will be 20°F lower than the thermostat temperature—the probiotics are retained. A great way to preserve your harvest without turning on the stove!

1/2 cup kefir
1 cup pureed fruit (Blenheim apricot, raspberries, plum, etc.)

1. Combine kefir and fruit in high-speed blender or food processor and blend until well combined.

2. Taste. If it tastes rather sweet, add a bit more kefir. The sweetness will be stronger as the leather dehydrates.

3. Spread on paraflex sheets and place on dehydrator trays or alternatively place on parchment paper on trays and set into dehydrator at 115°F for 8 to 12 hours.

4. When leather easily peels and is not sticky, it is done. Peel and store in glass container for storage.

Yogurt

Yogurt is an excellent probiotic. However, it is different from kefir. Yogurt contains transient beneficial bacteria that keep the digestive system clean and provide food for the friendly bacteria that reside there. But kefir can actually colonize the intestinal tract, a feat that yogurt cannot match.

Yogurt still deserves a place as a worthwhile probiotic and ferment, and it can lend much flavor and enjoyment to your meals. Homemade yogurt is a much more powerful ferment than most store bought yogurts for two main reasons. First, by providing an anaerobic fermentation environment and storage in a glass container produces and retains more active LAB bacteria. Second, homemade yogurt is fermented for much longer than the 4 to 6 hour ferments of commercial brands. Commercial yogurt is often sold in plastic containers, allowing a free passage of air into the yogurt, resulting in LAB dying off before you get to consume it. The one to two companies selling yogurt in glass jars with screw top lids is an improvement, but it's not airtight. Plan to eat your yogurt within the first few days of making it to receive the highest probiotic benefit.

Longer ferment time means less lactose is left and this results in a lower-sugar content and more tolerance for lactose-intolerant systems.

Read the section on "Choosing Milk" on page 49 in the Dairy Kefir section.

Your homemade yogurt may not be as thick as what you find in the store especially if you are used to purchasing goat milk yogurt. Many yogurts have some odd additives to make them thicker. I've seen cornstarch, guar gum, and tapioca. Personally, I prefer to eat yogurt with just milk and cultures as the ingredients.

Yogurt serving ideas

- Eat as is!
- Add some savory seasonings such a salt, dill, or cinnamon.
- Yogurt can usually be easily substituted where kefir or sour cream is used. Be sure to see page 51 and the "Salad, Dressing and Dip" on page 81 for more ideas.

Using whey

Whey is full of protein, minerals and enzymes. Whey from fully fermented milk no longer contains lactose, and with its dose of probiotic organisms will help maintain a synergistic balance of the inner flora and encourage repair of gut dysbiosis. Whey also contains a fair number of minerals, particularly potassium, and a notable amount of vitamins, especially B2.

<u>Note</u>: Do not use whey as a starter for any vegetable ferment!

Here are a few ideas on how to use it:

- Drink it!
- Add to smoothies
- Freeze into ice cubes and blend them into smoothies for a more slushy texture or to cool-down a beverage on a hot day.
- Soak grains or replace water with whey when cooking them. Note: The probiotics will not survive high heat.
- Make popsicles
- Add to salad dressings or to thin thick dips

Yogurt Cheese and Whey

These are useful items to have on hand. This is essentially yogurt drained liquid (whey), and the end result is yogurt cheese. This process works with kefir, too!

Yields 1/3 yogurt cheese to 2/3 whey.

1 quart yogurt
Salt and or herbs if desired

1. Line a colander or sieve with tightly woven cheesecloth or dish towel.

2. Set the colander over a bowl, and scoop the yogurt into the cheesecloth. Make sure the whey dripping off is relatively thin and clear. If it's thick and white, you are losing too much "curd" and need more layers of cheesecloth.

3. Let yogurt drain for 6 to 24 hours, depending on the desired cheese thickness; the longer it drains, the thicker the resulting "cheese" will be. At room temperature, the yogurt will drain faster. In the fridge, the yogurt will drain overnight.

4. Tie up the cheesecloth/towel with the yogurt left inside and gently tie the sack to a wooden spoon placed across a container to catch even more whey. Store the finished products (whey and cheese) in glass containers in the refrigerator. To reuse the cheesecloth, simply rinse out and hang to dry.

5. Blend cheese with herbs and salt or use as a base for dips, dressings, or a plain spread. It tastes similar to cream cheese without all the junk added.

Raw Milk Yogurt

1-Liter Pickl-It

To save time, scale the recipe to make enough yogurt for the week.

> **1 quart raw whole milk**
> **1 to 2 tablespoons whole milk yogurt with cultures**
> **Thermometer**
> **Dehydrator, seedling heat pad or other method to maintain 95°F**

1. Gently heat milk to 95°F in a pot. Be careful not to overheat.

2. Add milk to Pickl-It jar and stir in yogurt gently.

3. Close lid and add airlock with water.

4. Using an Excalibur dehydrator with the trays removed, I can place the yogurt jar and set the temperature at 95°F. Alternatively, try using the lowest setting on your oven with the door a bit ajar.

5. Keep at this temperature for 12 hours and turn off heat. Leave at room temperature for up to 8 hours, checking to see if the yogurt has thickened. It will thicken more in the fridge.

6. Store in the fridge until ready to serve.

Starches

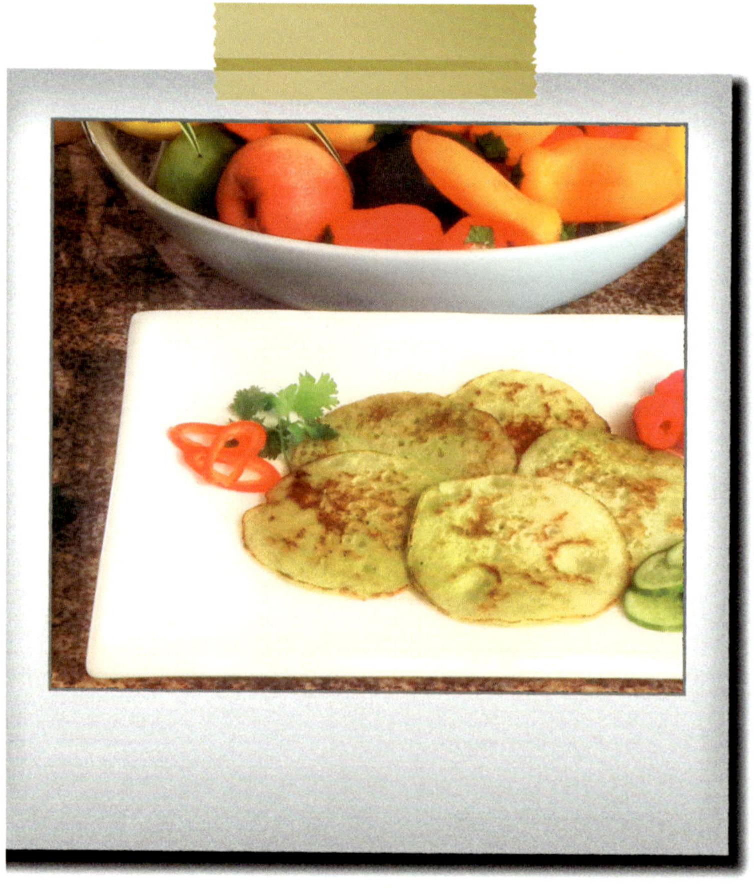

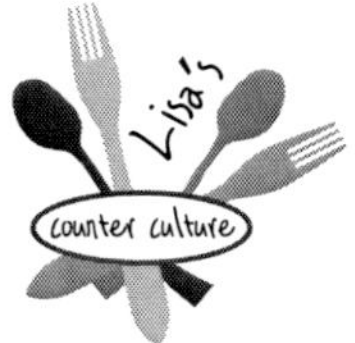

Starches

Dosa

Dosa are a thin, savory crepe-like flatbread. They are often described as a "pancake""
and are made of a batter of lentils and rice. Because dosa batter is lactofermented, it
tastes tangy and similar to sourdough.

Soaking and then fermenting the rice and lentils decrease the phytic acid. Phytase
is the enzyme that deactivates phytate, and it is quite active during fermentation.
In grains that contain high amounts of phytase, like wheat, rye, and buckwheat
(technically a pseudo-cereal, and gluten-free), a day of fermentation deactivates
most of the phytate. To degrade the phytate in low-phytase grains, however, the
fermentation time must be extended to 48 hours.

Fermentation reduces lectin load across the board, but it takes time. In lentils (not a
grain, but with similar antinutrient issues), 72 and 96 hours of fermentation at 107°F
eliminates 98% and 97.8% of the lectins, respectively. Overall, fermentation appears
to be pretty effective at reducing lectins (and cooking reduces them further).

Most dosa are made from black lentils, which have a black skin. The skin is steamed-
free and, generally, only the underlying creamy-ivory colored lentil is sold.

Dosa is typically a breakfast food, but we prefer to use them as a handy wrap for
whatever we are craving. From carnitas to scrambled eggs to leftover veggies—there
are endless options for fillings.

Idli rice is parboiled which makes the starches and sugars more easily available to
the lactic acid bacteria of the lentils. There are certain types of rice that do better at
idli/dosa fermentation than others. Jasmine or Basmati rice will work, but they are
different than the more traditional idli rice. Idli rice is better fuel for the LAB. Other
rice varieties will work, of course, but it was traditional to parboil the rice, preparing
it for the fermentation. Raw brown rice was not traditional.

Tips to successful dosa

Temperature: Dosa batter prefers temperatures above 75°F. I find the best results when the temperature is in the eighties. Since my home is usually cool and downright cold in winter, I discovered two great workarounds. My favorite is the seedling heat pad (see page 131). This device is great for warming your warmth-hungry ferments (like kefir and dosa). It raises the ambient room temperature 15 to 20 degrees. Another option is to use your dehydrator if you can remove the trays to leave a space for your Pickl-It. This works great with my Excalibur, then I set it at the lowest temperature of about 90°F.

Blending the batter

Best option: Scrape the soaking liquid, lentils, rice and salt/spices and blend to smooth using a high-speed blender (Blendtec or Vitamix).

Alternative: Drain the lentils and rice and reserve the soaking water. First, blend the rice and lentils well using a food processor and then add back the water with salt and seasonings to smooth.

Batter thickness: An easy pourable batter similar to a crepe or thin pancake batter works best for getting a thin dosa. You may need to add filtered water to your batter and mix it to get the right consistency.

Choosing a dosa pan

Here are two good options:

1. I prefer to use a Scanpan. It is non-stick, 100% PFOA free. The patented ceramic-titanium nonstick surface allows for high-heat cooking including searing, browning and deglazing, features not normally associated with nonstick cookware. Plus, it offers fool-proof food release and easy cleanup. I feel this is a safe pan to use for our family.

    With this pan, you can pour your batter in at room temperature and spread it thinly into a circle by swirling the pan. You don't need to add ghee at this point but I usually add a little and than more on top when I flip it.

    I love these pans! They are super easy to use and a breeze to clean.

2. Cast iron flat pan or frying pan: Heat pan and add a good bit of fat (ghee, coconut oil, or lard). When water "bounces" across surface, you're ready add the batter. Spoon about a 1/4 cup of dosa batter onto hot pan, using the back of the spoon, to a 6-inch diameter.

Red Lentil Dosa

1-Liter Pickl-It for one batch but I always double it and use a 1.5-Liter or 2-Liter jar.

Red lentils, which are often easier to locate in your local grocery, create a beautiful reddish-pink batter. Don't skip the turmeric—it's worth finding organic turmeric—as science has shown it offers numerous healthy properties, in addition to a pleasing flavor.

> **3/4 cup Idli rice**
> **1/4 cup red lentils**
> **1 cup warm water**
> **5 grams salt**
> **1/2 teaspoon ground turmeric**
> **Organic ghee for frying and drizzling**

1. Place rice and lentils and water in a Pickl-It. Cover and add airlock with water. Allow mixture to soak for 12 to 24 hours at room temperature. Drain, reserving the soaking water.

2. Rinse Pickl-It jar with filtered water and set aside.

3. Place rice and lentils in food processor. Blend until smooth. Add reserved soaking water and blend with rice/lentils. Stir in salt and turmeric. Scrape the pureed rice/lentils back into the Pickl-It, cover, and lock lid. Add airlock with water. Ferment for 24 to 48 hours away from light.

4. Heat cast iron flat pan. Brush on a thick layer of ghee. When water "bounces," you're ready to add the batter. Spoon about a 1/4 cup of dosa batter onto hot pan, using the back of the spoon, to a 6-inch diameter. If using a scan pan, see directions page 60.

5. Cook for 1 to 1.5 minutes. Drizzle top with melted ghee.

6. Using a long, thin spatula, loosen baked edge, then slide spatula under entire dosa, "releasing" it from the pan; lift and flip, cooking additional minute until light-golden brown.

The batter stores up to 7 days in a well-sealed glass container—preferably a Pickl-It with a Plug'R. Before cooking, remove the batter from the refrigerator, allowing it to warm up to room temperature, before cooking.

Variations: Add 4 tablespoons grated coconut, 1 tablespoon grated fresh ginger and 1 finely chopped chili to the batter just before cooking.

Urad Gota Dosa

1-Liter Pickl-It for one batch, but I always double it and use the 1.5-Liter or 2-Liter jar. This recipe is a bit more traditional and our favorite.

Fenugreek attracts the same type of wild yeast as the urad gota. Traditionally, the seeds are put in the rice pan and lentil pan so that both the urad dal and the rice draw wild yeast. Also, fenugreek is helpful for nursing mothers in encouraging lactation. Fenugreek has numerous health benefits including aid in digestion (organicfacts.net/health-benefits/vegetable/health-benefits-of-fenugreek.html)

3/4 cup Idli rice
1/4 cup urad dal
1 cup warm water
5 grams salt
1/4 teaspoon ground fenugreek
Organic ghee for frying and drizzling

1. Place rice, lentils and water in a "Pickl-It." Cover and add airlock (fill with water). Allow mixture to soak for 24 hours at room temperature. Drain, reserving the soaking water.

2. Rinse Pickl-It jar with filtered water and set aside.

3. Place rice and lentils in food processor. Blend until smooth. Add reserved soaking water and blend with rice/lentils. Stir in salt and fenugreek. Scrape the pureed rice/lentils back into the Pickl-It, cover, and lock lid. Add airlock with water. Ferment for 24 to 48 hours away from light.

4. Heat cast iron flat pan and brush on thick layer of ghee. When water "bounces" across surface, you're ready to cook dosa. With 1/4-cup ladle, spoon dosa batter onto hot pan, using the back of the ladle, to a 6-inch diameter. For scan pan, follow the directions on page 60.

5. Cook for 1 to 1.5 minutes. Drizzle top with melted ghee.

6. Using a long, thin spatula, loosen baked edge, then slide spatula under entire dosa, "releasing" it from the pan; lift and flip, cooking an additional minute until light-golden brown.

The batter stores up to 7 days in a well-sealed glass container, preferably a Pickl-It with a Plug'R. Before cooking, remove the batter from the refrigerator, allowing it to warm up to room temperature, before cooking.

Variations: 2 tablespoons of chopped fresh cilantro (not traditional but delicious)Add 4 tablespoons grated coconut, 1 tablespoon grated fresh ginger and 1 finely chopped chili to the batter just before cooking.

Potato and Sweet Potato

Amazingly, if you study traditional preparations of tubers like potatoes and sweet potatoes, you'll discover a method of preparation that made them much more digestible. The answer is soaking and fermenting! Another bonus, with a little planning, this is easily done at home with delicious results.

Another benefit of soaking potatoes is the reduction or almost elimination of acrylamide. Kathleen Mills, the owner of Pickl-It, has this information on the website:

> *"Acrylamide is formed by a heat-induced reaction between sugar (glucose, fructose and sucrose) and asparagine. Known as the Maillard reaction, this process is responsible for the brown colour and tasty flavour of baked, fried and toasted foods." Food Quality News*

> *In 2002, the European factory-food industry was shaken by the discovery of acrylamide, described as "a neuro-toxin, genome-affecting, possible carcinogenic compound", created during the baking of gingerbread.*

> *Over the next few years, other high-starch foods—French fries, chips, pan-fries, latkes, and even some canned black olives—were also found to contain questionable levels of acrylamide. (Friedman 2003; Dybing and others 2005)*

> *"Acrylamide formation in potato tubers is mainly determined by the contents of glucose, fructose and not by the content of the asparagine."*
> *—Amrein*

> *As spontaneous, natural fermentation methods reduce the potatoes' glucose and fructose, acrylamide formation will be disrupted.*

> *Unlike an open-bowl water-only soaking-method which leaves a thick residue of starch in the bottom of the bowl, there will be no starch in the Pickl-It (Pickl-It.com).*

> *That's because the Pickl-It environment supports a healthy community of lactic acid bacteria, which are very efficient at breaking down and reducing sugars and the starch, leaving only clear brine and not undigested starch-sludge.*

Fermented fries won't burn, and the tendency to get gassy from potatoes is also reduced greatly.

If you want to further reduce the acrylamide and sugar/starches, then add a broad-spectrum starter to reduce acrylamide by 98%. Using the Pickl-It without the Caldwell starter yields about an 84% reduction. (Caldwell's vegetable starter is the only one available that is made from organic veggies). Note that using whey or the Body Ecology starter (a narrow-spectrum starter—similar to what is used by the food industry based in dairy bacteria) are less than 50%. See "Appendix B: Food Resources" on page 133 for finding the Caldwell starter.

Healthy Fries

Courtesy of Kathleen Mills, Pickl-It. Modified slightly.

Potatoes (sweet, yukon, russet or fingerlings)
Salt
Water
Fat (bacon, ghee, coconut oil or ghee)
Caldwell starter (optional)

1. Cut potatoes into thick or thin fries (or shred, slice, or dice). Place in the Pickl-It and add a 3.5% salt brine. Close the lid and add water to the airlock.

2. Caldwell starter: Each Caldwell packet is adequate for 4.5 pounds of food. For 3 pounds of potatoes, use 1/2 a packet in a 3.5% brine. Dissolve the starter in some water, then add to the brine.

3. Ferment for 24 to 48 hours. Note that a shorter ferment time is needed as more surface area of the potato is exposed (shredded will be much shorter than whole potatoes).

4. Drain your potatoes and toss the brine.

5. Coat the potatoes with your favorite fat (bacon grease, duck, lard or coconut oil) and favorite herbs (rosemary, thyme) and/or spices.

6. Bake at 350°F for 35-45 minutes, depending on how thick or thin the fries are.

Note: Try to ferment your potatoes when possible. At the very least, soak them for a minimum of 6 hours in a salt brine. This is a traditional potato preparation method. Fermented potatoes can also be used to make mashed, roasted and other typical potato dishes.

Happy Belly Buckwheat Pancakes

Modified slightly from Chris Kresser's recipe. This recipe requires a little planning, but I find the batter is good for a few days after it is prepared.

Buckwheat is not in the wheat family and is actually a fruit seed that is related to rhubarb and sorrel, making it a suitable substitute for grains for people who are sensitive to wheat or other grains that contain protein glutens.

1 cup buckwheat groats (raw, not toasted)
A few tablespoons yogurt or kefir
1.5 cups water
1 cup fresh yogurt or kefir
2 eggs beaten
1/2 cup milk (or unsweetened almond milk or water)
1 teaspoon baking soda
1 teaspoon vanilla
Pinch of salt

1. The night before cooking, combine the buckwheat groats, a few tablespoons of kefir or yogurt and 1.5 cups of filtered water in a glass bowl and stir.

2. Leave covered at room temperature for 12 to 24 hours.

3. After soaking, rinse yogurt/water from buckwheat.

4. Put buckwheat in a blender with one cup of fresh yogurt. The amount you use depends on how thick you'd like the pancakes to be. Blend until smooth.

5. Add the rest of the ingredients and blend.

6. Put a cast iron or heavy ceramic (e.g., Le Crueset) pan or Scan pan (my personal favorite) on the burner over medium-to-medium high heat and let the pan heat.

7. The secret to cooking pancakes is to make sure the pan gets hot before you add the batter. I use my scan pan—so I don't need to use much fat for cooking. I melt the butter on top.

8. Make sure the pan is hot and add a generous amount of fat (ghee, coconut oil, lard, etc.) to the pan. When fat is shimmering, ladle pancake batter into the pan. Allow pancakes to cook almost all the way through before flipping. You can either continue to add fat before each new pancake or not. With more fat, the pancakes are almost like fritters; with less fat, they are more like typical pancakes.

9. Top with fruit and butter if desired.

Ferment Companions

Beverages

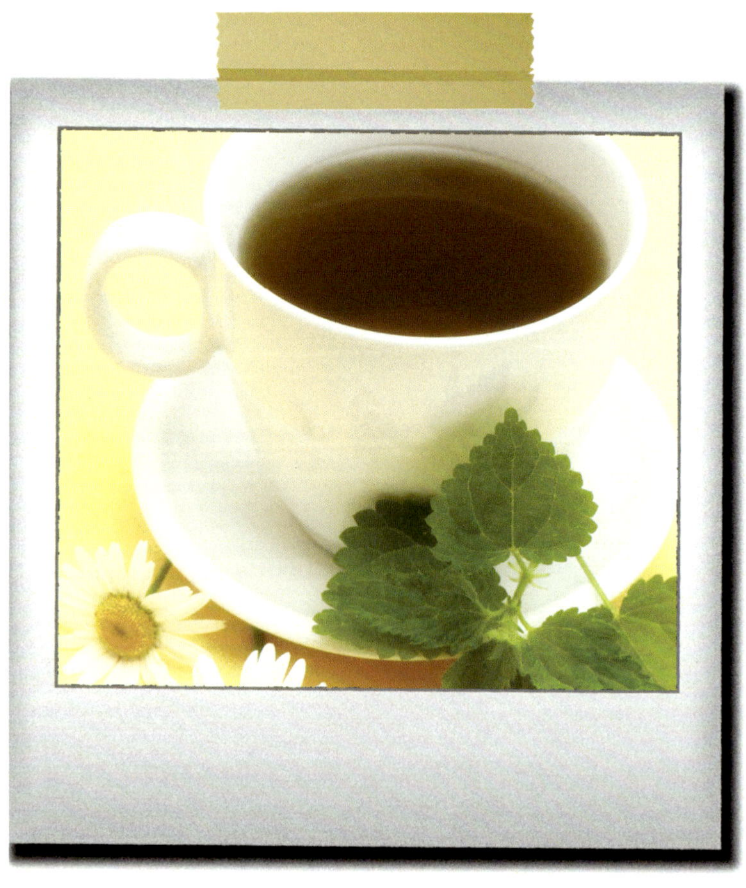

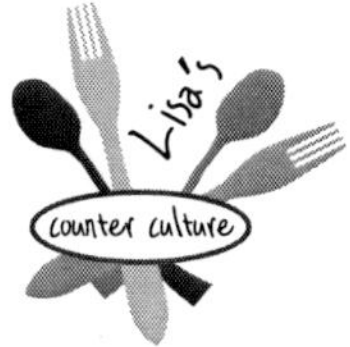

Beverages

I've included just a few of my more unusual and often requested beverage recipes in this section. These are all nourishing and healing drinks, but they are not fermented. Be sure to see Fermented Beverages on page 11.

Stinging Nettle Tea

I love this tea, and you can cook the leftover greens afterwards! Stinging nettles are often considered a weed, but they are definitely worth eating for their nutritional and healing properties. Plus, they are delicious!

Here's why you should try them. Research has shown that this plant boasts notable levels of vitamins A and C as well as health-boosting minerals like calcium, magnesium, iron, potassium, phosphorous, manganese, iodine, and sulfur.

And the sting? As soon as the plant is simmered or steamed, the stinging hairs are now harmless. Be sure to wear thick gloves when handling. I discovered stinging nettles at a local farmer's market one spring, but I later had to plant my own to sustain my new found love. Be sure to plant in a pot. Like mint, they can quickly take over.

Large handful fresh stinging nettles
10 ounces boiling water
Squeeze of fresh lemon (optional)

1. Carefully place nettles into a small pot. Boil some water and then pour over the nettles.

2. Let sit for 10 minutes. Strain and drink. Add lemon squeeze to make it even better.

3. Save greens and saute with garlic and ghee or your favorite fat. These are worth eating!

Supertonic

Keep The Yuckies Away!

This recipe is easy to put together. Use equal parts of all ingredients, except for apple cider vinegar. These ingredients should be as fresh as possible and preferably organic. Use dried herbs in an emergency.

> **Organic raw apple cider vinegar**
> **1 part fresh chopped garlic cloves**
> **1 part fresh chopped white/yellow onion**
> **1 part fresh chopped hot peppers (jalapeno)**
> **1 part fresh grated ginger root**
> **1 part fresh grated horseradish root**

1. Shred all ingredients (except the vinegar) through a food processor or by hand.

2. Take caution when grating the fresh horseradish. When shredding, the fumes can be quite powerful.

3. Fill a glass jar 3/4 of the way full with equal parts by volume of the above chopped and grated ingredients.

4. Fill the jar with raw vinegar.

5. Close and shake vigorously. Then top off the vinegar if necessary. I keep mine closed up in the cupboard.

6. Shake or stir once a day for two weeks, then filter the mixture through a clean cloth or fine meshed strainer. Compost the leftovers.

7. Store in a dark colored glass bottle at room temperature. This will last a long time. It even improves over time.

Note: I believe this tonic originated from Dr. Richard Schutze. The tonic is extremely powerful as it comes from all fresh ingredients. It is touted as a modern day plague tonic. Don't underestimate its power. I would start slowly, only taking a little bit from the tincture bottle, especially if you want to give it to your kids.

Regular dosage is 0.5 to 1 oz. once, twice, or more times a day. (You can dilute with water if you feel it is too strong.)

Real Ginger Tea

I never much cared for ginger tea until I had some made from fresh ginger. It's a very healing tea when you are a bit under the weather or have a sore throat (add honey).

> **1 tablespoon fresh ginger grated (easy with a microplane)**
> **1 cup hot water**
> **Lemon squeeze and/or raw honey (optional)**

1.   Pour hot water over ginger and steep for 10 minutes.

2.   Strain and add lemon/honey if desired. Enjoy!

Green Juice

Makes 8 ounces.

I love to start the day with some juiced green veggies. Unlike most recipes I come across, my basic combo is low on sugar. Since I do need to watch my blood sugar, I do my best to keep this more savory than sweet.

If your produce looks tired, then juicing them won't yield the same benefits as happy, fresh produce. Also choosing a juicer that is efficient at getting every last drop out of greens is more economical in the long run. I love my Omega 8000 juicer. You can find out more about juicers on page 131.

> **Large handful of Kale/chard/parsley/cilantro)**
> **1 clove garlic**
> **1/4 carrot or 1/2 small peeled beet or both if greens are rather bitter**
> **2 small cucumbers (pickling size)**
> **Celery (70 % volume)**

1.   Wash and cut veggies to fit into juicer. (Slower juicing results in less oxidation and foam.)

2.   Take the time to breath and anticipate all those healing nutrients entering your system. Enjoy!

Tips

- Reconsider spinach. I don't typically juice spinach—I find it hard to digest unless cooked with some fat.
- Reserve odds and ends from prepping salad, preparing veggies for side dishes to juice that day. Cucumber ends, broccoli stems, etc.

Broth & Soup

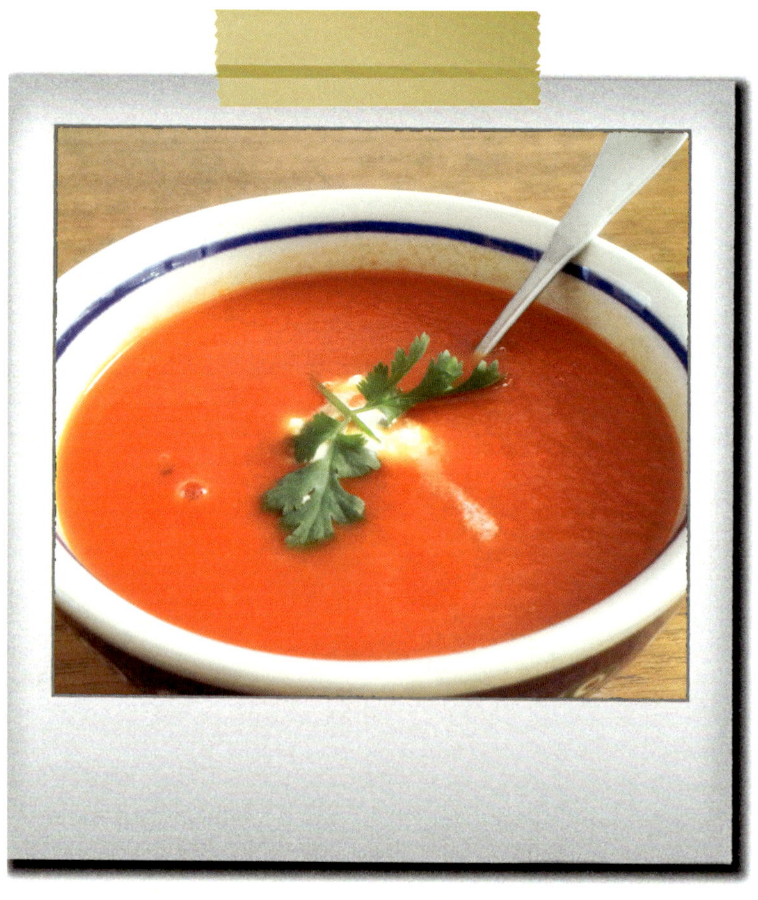

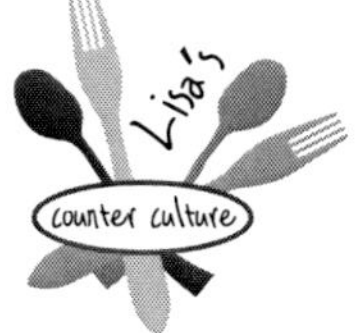

Broth & Soup

Soups are one of my most favorite meals. I find them comforting and always a crowd-pleaser with my family. We all love soup! Good soup can easily make the best use of what is offered seasonally, so you never get bored. Homemade stock and bone broth is much more nutritious, economical and tastier. It's so simple and easy, once you learn a few tips. Broth and stock are ideal ways to stock your freezer. Make a lot and save time later, and you'll always have a quick remedy on hand when feeling under the weather. Commercial broth is not simmered long enough to extract all the components of this healthful food, and canning renders it a dead food in my opinion.

Bone broth is a good calcium source, especially relevant if you are avoiding dairy-based foods. Bone broth provides our bodies with bioavailable (very easy to consume, digest and absorb) forms of calcium, magnesium, phosphorous and other trace minerals that are so lacking in our diets today due to depleted soils and high volumes of refined food consumption. (Source: wapf.org)

From *Nourishing Traditions*, page 116:

> *Meat and fish stocks are used almost universally in traditional cuisines—French, Italian, Chinese, Japanese, African, South American, Middle Eastern and Russian; but the use of homemade meat broths to produce nourishing and flavorful soups and sauces has almost completely disappeared from the American culinary tradition.*

Properly prepared meat stocks are extremely nutritious, containing the minerals of bone, cartilage, marrow and vegetables as electrolytes, a form that is easy to assimilate. Acidic wine or vinegar added during cooking helps draw minerals, particularly calcium, magnesium and potassium, into the broth. Dr. Francis Pottenger, author of the famous cat studies as well as articles on the benefits of gelatin in broth, taught that the stockpot was the most important piece of kitchen equipment to have.

According to the September/October 2011 Well Being Journal's *"Bone Broth Delivers Minerals & Macro Nutrients"* article, these are the minerals and nutrients in bone broth soup:

Loads of calcium, phosphorus, magnesium and potassium

Gelatin: Long slow simmering of bone broth makes it a gelatinous substance. Gelatin helps with digestibility, soothes the intestinal lining, can decrease respiratory problems, allergies and colic. It is known for therapeutic support for those with ulcers, diabetes, muscle diseases, bone problems, infections and even cancer.

Amino acids glycine and proline: Glycine helps with liver detoxification, wound healing and any condition requiring rapid growth such as pregnancy. Proline is part of connective tissue and is an important amino acid for people with tissue and joint problems.

Hyaluronic acid: This acid is a "colloid." It attracts gastric juices to the surface of food, helping with digestion. Most foods repel gastric juices, impairing digestion.

All the components that make up connective tissue: The most important component is chondroitin sulfate. This is commonly sold as an expensive supplement for joint problems. Chondroitin sulfate is free with homemade bone broth.

What's the difference between bone broth and stock? Not much. If bones/ meat are missing, then this is referred to as stock. Or if bone broth is filtered to just the liquid and then used as a base for another preparation, then it's a stock. If other ingredients are added, then the term soup may be used. It's the bones that create the magic, and the results are delicious!

Bone broth, like most traditional foods, is the most nutritious when they are sourced from the best circumstances. Ideally, grassfed pastured animals that are humanely raised, organic seasonal vegetables, sustainable are all key concepts that led to the best results.

Using stocks and broths

- Drink like tea with every meal or as a snack
- Cook rice/grains with broth to add minerals and flavor
- Make soups
- Reduction sauces
- Gravies
- Use to braise vegetables or over potatoes/rice
- Use to make chawanmushi! My favorite Japanese comfort food—savory egg custard

Oxtail Bone Broth

Oxtails or bison tails make the best stock because they provide everything you need: stock, gel, cartilage and tendons, meat, and fat. And oh, do they give flavor.

If you choose to brown the oxtails before you make the broth, then this will intensify the flavor and the color. But you can skip this step if you are pressed for time. I like to throw the oxtail into a pan and roast it at 350°F for an hour. Or you can brown it—melt tallow, lard or butter and brown all sides of the oxtail. Scrape all juices and fat into your cooking pot.

Note: It's best to add salt to taste before serving.

> **2 pounds oxtail or bison tail, cut into 1 inch pieces**
> **3 carrots, scrubbed and coarsely chopped**
> **3 celery ribs, coarsely chopped**
> **1 medium onion, coarsely chopped**
> **Handful garlic cloves**
> **¼ cup organic apple cider vinegar**
> **Filtered water to cover**

1. Place bones, vegetables into slow cooker or large Dutch oven.

2. Cover with filtered water.

3. Add apple cider vinegar.

4. Let sit for 1 hour (draws out the minerals and vitamins from the bones)

5. Bring to simmer or cook on high for slow cooker–skim any scum that rises– lower heat to maintain a simmer.

6. Cook for at least 12 hours and as long as 72 hours

7. Strain and cool. Reserve the meat and discard the vegetables. Chop the meat and fat and tendons and keep in a bowl or container while the stock cools. (Note: this step may take several hours or overnight in order to allow the fat to cool and harden.)

8. When the stock has cooled, take off the layer of fat and reserve for cooking (or adding back in to the oxtail soup when you make it.)

9. Store broth in smaller containers for freezer if desired.

Chicken Bone Broth

This is how my Polish grandmother taught me to make this. You can also stick to the recipe in *Nourishing Traditions* (page 124). I have merged my grandmother's recipe a bit with the one from *Nourishing Traditions*.

Try to get a smaller bony chicken, which makes the best stock. Three pounds is ideal. Feet are a great way to get gelatin and flavor into your broth.

One chicken including back, neck and feet
2 tablespoons apple cider vinegar
1 large onion halved
2 carrots
2 ribs celery
1 parsnip
Several to many cloves garlic
Fresh parsley
1 teaspoon peppercorns
Several mushrooms

1. Cut chicken into several pieces.

2. Place chicken into large stainless steel stock pot with vinegar; water, all veggies—except the parsley.

3. Let stand for 30 minutes to one hour.

4. Bring to boil, remove scum and simmer for 6 to 24 hours. Longer leads to more gelatin, minerals and flavor.

5. Add parsley 15 minutes before serving.

6. Serve as soup or reserve chicken meat for other preparations.

7. Strain broth, cool and store in fridge or freezer.

Note: For a clearer stock or if your chicken source is not ideal, remove the skin before cooking.

Variations: Stir in a beaten egg into simmering broth and garnish with parsley/cilantro. Simmer some broth with a slice of ginger for 5 minutes. Add two teaspoons of miso when warm (not boiling) and a dash of fish sauce, and top with scallions.

Basic Bone Broth

Bones (mix marrow and knuckle bones 3 to 4 pounds)
1/4 cup organic raw apple cider vinegar
1 onion
2 to 3 carrots
2 to 3 ribs celery
1 teaspoon peppercorn
Garlic (optional)
Parsley/kale

1. Place bones in a very large pot or slow cooker.

2. Cover with filtered water

3. Let sit for 1 hour (draws out the minerals and vitamins from the bones)

4. Bring to simmer or cook on high in slow cooker. Skim any scum that rises. Lower heat to maintain a simmer.

5. Cook for at least 12 hours and as long as 72 hours

6. Add another 1/2 bunch of kale and 1/2 bunch of parsley.

7. Strain and cool. Reserve all the meat and discard the vegetables. Chop the meat, fat and tendons and keep in a bowl or container while the stock cools. (This may take several hours or overnight in order to allow the fat to cool and harden).

8. When the stock has cooled, take off the layer of fat and reserve for cooking or leave on to seal broth for the freezer (or to add back into the soup when you make it).

9. Store broth in smaller containers for freezing if desired.

Note: Replenish the water as it evaporates. Add a little water every day as needed.

Quick Cheat Fish Stock

Just takes about 15 minutes!

> **1 to 2 pounds cleaned mussels, clams or cockles in shell or shrimp shells**
> **Filtered water**
> **Dash sherry (optional)**
> **Salt, pepper and spices (parsley, cilantro and/or lemongrass)**
> **Clove garlic crushed**
> **Tablespoon of butter or dash olive oil at end**

1. Place all ingredients in a small stock pot, cover with water. Turn heat to high and close lid.

2. Shake occasionally to stir up the pot. Shellfish should start to open in 5 to 7 minutes Thicker shell clams take longer and larger shells take longer than small ones. As soon as shells all open, they are ready to serve. Careful not to overcook to avoid rubbery shellfish.

Optional: Before serving, add a tablespoon of butter or olive oil. Or add some coconut milk and a pinch of saffron.

Note: Shrimp shell stock takes about 20 minutes to cook at a gentle boil.

Cream of Any Vegetable Soup

Very easy and basic—cook/roast vegetable with flavorings

> **2 cups chopped cooked vegetables**
> **2 cups broth**
> **¼ cup cream, sour cream or yogurt (adds probiotics!)**

1. Blend and heat.

2. Adjust seasonings. Add blended cooked rice or potato for a thicker soup.

Note: Cultured cream (sour cream, piima creme or creme fraiche) is important for providing the enzymes and fat soluble vitamins needed for our bodies to use the minerals in the soup. Be sure to add the cream to your serving bowl when the soup has cooled slightly to preserve these heat sensitive nutrients.

Savory Simple Tomato Soup

Makes about 4 servings

A quick 10-minute soup. I find it very comforting, with good fats that satiate my appetite.

1 pint tomatoes pureed
1 clove garlic minced
2 thick slices of onion diced
2 to 3 tablespoons butter
Dash anchovy or fish sauce (optional)
½ cup sour cream
2 tablespoons cilantro and parsley (or basil)
Salt and pepper to taste

1. Sauté onion and garlic in butter over medium heat. Add tomatoes, salt, pepper, anchovy, cilantro and parsley and lower the heat.

2. Using an immersion blender and carefully blend the soup. Alternatively, remove mixture and blend in a blender/food processor and return to the pot.

3. Add two tablespoons butter and sour cream and gently warm through. Taste and adjust seasonings.

Almost Polish Pickle Soup

A great way to use extra pickles and juice and get bone broth in at the same time!

5 cups chicken broth
1/2 cup dill pickles finely chopped
1/2 cup pickle juice (dill)
2 tablespoons butter
1/2 cup onion finely minced
2 teaspoons minced garlic
3 teaspoons salt or to taste
1 tablespoon fresh dill chopped
1/2 teaspoon white pepper
1 teaspoon Red Boat fish sauce (optional for extra zip)
1/4 cup pureed potato to thicken (optional but delicious)
1 cup milk (warm)

1. Melt butter in a large stock pot over medium heat and saute onions.

2. Add chicken broth dill pickles, pickle juice, fish sauce and seasonings. Bring to a low simmer for 5 to 7 minutes.

3. Whisk in potatoes (if using). Remove from heat and whisk in milk.

4. Garnish with fresh dill and sour cream.

Salad, Dressing, and Dip

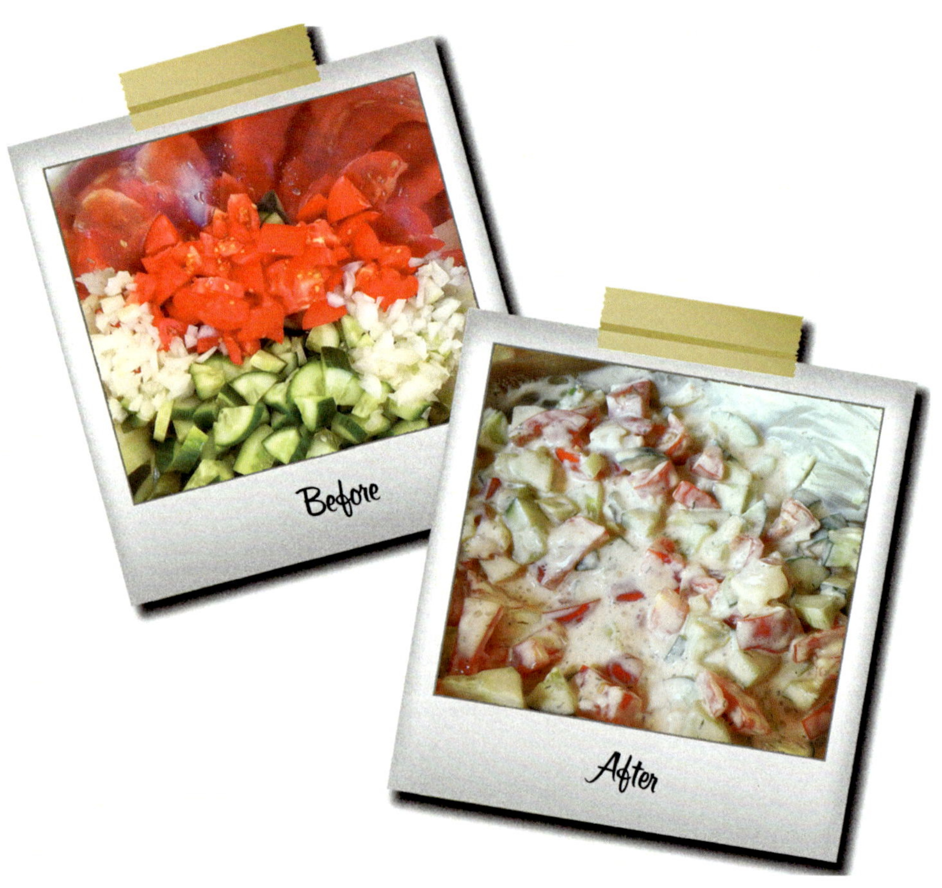

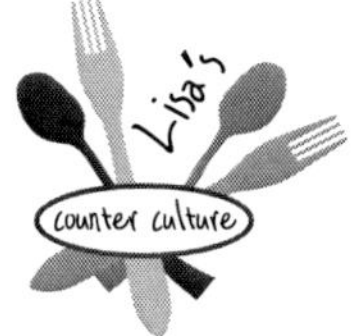

Salad, Dressing and Dip

Here are some of my "regulars" that I hope you will enjoy. Salad, dressing and dip are a wonderful chance to reflect the seasons. Summer dressings rely on summer herbs like basil and cilantro and purees of avocado or tomatoes. Spring is fava bean dip time! Feta cheese dip is a fall favorite. Salads fall into a similar pattern. Check your garden or local farmer's market for inspiration. Use what is freshest and local, unless you are crafty and can pull out preserved treasures from dehydrating, freezing or fermenting from a previous season.

Once you see how fast and easy it is to make your own dressings and dips, you will never be tempted by a commercial jar or bottle again! It's economical and quick and the taste can't be beat! All you need is some acid, a fat, and a small whisk (whisk is not really required). Herbs, spices and seasonings can add to the endless possible combinations. Plus, you'll know exactly what's in your dressing and dip versus the long paragraph of weird nonfood ingredients that appear on most commercial products.

Have a favorite store dressing? Read the ingredients and I bet you can quickly make a better, cleaner version in just minutes. This is true for dips and some salads, too.

A ratio of 3:1 for fat to acid is common, but I find that I like a 2:1 ratio. You will need to experiment a little to see what suits your taste best. Keep in mind that healthy fats like olive oil, coconut oil and even bacon fat are important for your system to be able to absorb nutrients from the salad greens and vegetables.

Acids: Apple cider vinegar, balsamic vinegar, kombucha vinegar and lemon juice are my personal favorites. And more vinegars: red wine, rice wine, sherry champagne, white wine, herb, fruit and seasoned vinegar.

Fats: Extra virgin olive oil is my main go-to, but sesame, avocado, walnut, macadamia and coconut oil are all great. Want a decadent treat? Try 3 tablespoons warm bacon fat whisked with 3 tablespoons of apple cider vinegar, 1/2 teaspoon of mustard, drop of honey, and salt /pepper over spinach salad with sliced hardboiled eggs and crisp bacon.

Add Ins: Dried or fresh herbs and spices, garlic, sour cream or yogurt, chili peppers, shallots or scallions, mustard, horseradish, fish sauce, honey, maple syrup, grated hard cheese, capers, olives, chutneys or a smidgen of jam.

Sprouted Quinoa Salad

One cup of quinoa makes at least 6 to 8 servings. This will get better sitting in the fridge for a few days.

> **1 cup quinoa sprouted (see note)**
> **2 cups total, chopped parsley, cilantro (or add mint/basil)**
> **1/4 cup diced red onion**
> **1 cup chopped tomatoes**
> **Salt and pepper to taste**
> **1/8 cup lemon juice**
> **1/4 cup olive oil**
> **Sheep or goat feta makes a great addition**

1. Take 1 cup sprouted quinoa and cover with boiling water.

2. Let quinoa soak for 35 minutes, then drain the water.

3. Mix with rest of ingredients and adjust to taste.

4. Refrigerate for at least an hour or more to let flavors deepen.

Note: Check your health food store or my amazon store on my website.

Summer Salad

I loved eating this as a kid in the summers, and it must be genetic since my kids adore this, too! I have made this with a smaller amount of red onion to keep it kid friendly. Feel free to add more to your liking.

> **2 cups chopped cucumbers**
> **2 cups chopped tomatoes or thinly sliced radishes**
> **1/2 to 3/4 cup sour cream**
> **3 tablespoons finely minced red or sweet onion**
> **2 cloves garlic crushed**
> **Salt and white pepper to taste (don't skimp on salt)**
> **Fresh chopped dill (optional)**

1. Combine all ingredients and taste. Adjust seasonings if needed.

2. Place in fridge for at least an hour to let juices and flavors deepen. (It's worth the wait.)

Miso Dressing

Makes enough to dress one large salad. You can also try garbanzo miso.

1 tablespoon miso
2 ounces olive oil
Clove garlic though garlic press or finely minced
Dash sesame oil
Several tablespoons apple cider vinegar or rice vinegar
Dash anchovy or fish sauce (optional)
Salt and pepper to taste

1. Add ingredients to cup and blend with a whisk.

2. Taste and adjust ingredients as needed.

Cultured Caesar Dressing

Super quick and wonderful.

3 to 4 tablespoons fermented mayonnaise
2 tablespoons fresh lemon juice
1 teaspoon Red Boat fish sauce
½ to 1 clove garlic finely minced or more to taste
Fresh pepper to taste

1. Whisk all ingredients together. Thin with water as needed.

Feta Cheese Dip

This is adapted from *How to Cook Everything* by Mark Bittman. Fermented sour cream and feta add some happy bacteria to this dish.

1 cup of goat or sheet feta
1 cup sour cream
2 tablespoons minced scallion
2 tablespoons fresh parsley minced
Garlic clove minced
1/2 teaspoon marjoram and/or oregano leaves
1/4 teaspoon thyme leaves dried
Fresh ground black (lots)
Salt to taste (may not need any due to salt in feta)
Splash lemon juice or apple cider vinegar

1. Combine all ingredients. Mash together for a more lumpy dip or use blender/ food processor for a smoother dip.

2. Adjust seasonings. Chill for 20 minutes prior to serving.

Fresh Fava Bean Dip

Fresh organic ingredients make this dip shine!

1 cup fresh fava beans
1/4 cup fresh cilantro
3 tablespoons tahini (Trader Joe's has a decent fresh tahini)
3 tablespoons lemon juice or apple cider vinegar (more to taste)
1 to 2 cloves minced garlic
1/4 teaspoon cumin
2 tablespoons extra virgin olive oil
White pepper to taste

1. Blanch fava beans for 5 to 7 minutes. (Blanch: Drop into boiling water and than remove to bowl of ice to cool). Remove fava skins if desired.

2. Blend fava beans with remaining ingredients until smooth. Adjust seasonings. Chill for 20 minutes prior to serving.

Serving suggestion: Wrap in Romaine or butter lettuce or serve as a dip with fresh veggies.

Artichoke Dip

Great with grilled fish or chicken. Try it with fresh veggies as well.

7 ounces marinated artichoke hearts
2/3 cup olive oil
1 cup Parmesan or Machego cheese grated
2 cloves garlic minced
Salt and pepper to taste

1. Blend with a food processor or high-speed blender until smooth.

2. Adjust seasonings if needed.

Main

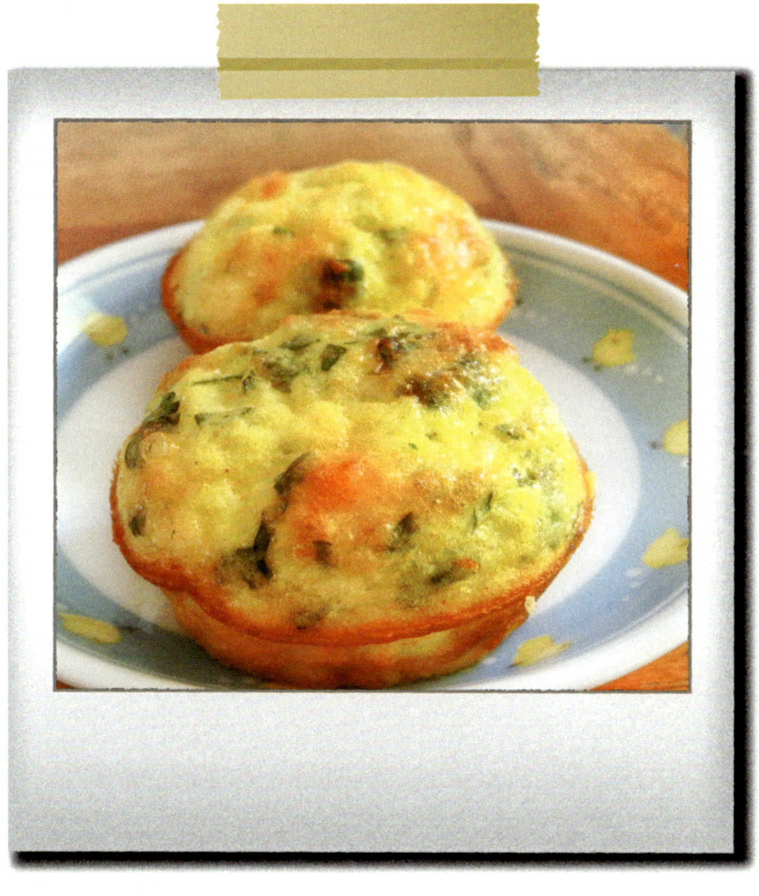

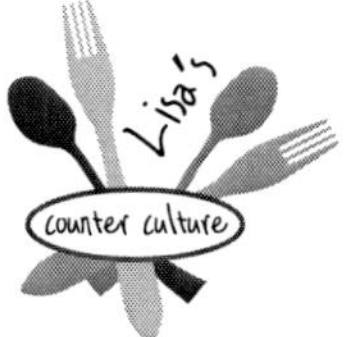

Eggs

Eggs are one of my main staples. There are endless ways to prepare them and the convenience of a simple hard-boiled egg is a wonderfully easy snack to take along anywhere.

Eggs are made of high-quality proteins and essential fat-soluble vitamins, particularly vitamins A and D. They are also a valuable source of special long-chain fatty acids (EPA and DHA), which are important for the development of the nervous system of children as well as maintaining mental acuity for adults. This is a true "brain food."

Eggs also provide one of the most concentrated sources of choline (a type of B vitamin needed to keep cholesterol moving in the blood stream).

One egg provides 13 essential nutrients, all in the yolk (contrary to popular belief, the yolk is far higher in nutrients than the white). Eggs are rich in iodine, for making thyroid hormones, and phosphorus, essential for healthy bones and teeth.

Of course, egg quality is a concern. Studies show that commercially-raised eggs are up to 19 times higher in pro-inflammatory omega-6 fatty acids. Unfortunately, almost all eggs sold in supermarkets—even the organic eggs sold at chains such as Whole Foods and Wild Oats—are not truly pasture-raised. To find these eggs, check your local farmer's market or visit the Eat Wild website to locate a source in your area.

Keep in mind, even when paying top dollar for high quality eggs from pastured chickens or other poultry, eggs are one of the least expensive sources of complete protein.

Think you may have an intolerance to eggs? (If you have a serious egg allergy, don't try this without first consulting your doctor.) Try duck or quail eggs or eggs from chickens not fed on soy and/or corn. I know many folks who are able to eat and enjoy these alternatives without any digestive issues. Yolks are also much better tolerated than whites for people with sensitivities.

Duck eggs are amazing. They are richer in flavor, and the whites are more viscous or stretchy than chicken eggs—a quality that does a great and better job of holding and binding food together than previously relied on flour or grains. I love duck eggs in crustless quiche or in meatloaf. They are also a bit larger with thicker shells than chicken eggs, so a bit more effort is needed to crack. Try them and see what you think. It's nice to have some variety. I have also had peacock and goose eggs, but duck eggs are my favorite.

I don't recommend eating raw egg whites from fresh eggs. Yolks are fine since they contain avidin, which interferes with the absorption of biotin and also contain trypsin inhibitors, which interfere with protein digestion. These are not problems when eggs are cooked.

Truly fresh organic eggs from pastured chickens look and taste different to what many of us have become used to eating. When cracked, the yolk should be a dark deep yellow and sit high and round on top of the white. It's hard to go back to factory-farmed eggs once you've had fresh! Also, keep in mind that eggs are a seasonal food. If your source of eggs does not decrease in the winter, that may be a clue that their chickens are not truly pastured (unless you live near the equator). Egg production naturally decreases during the colder seasons and when the days are shorter since egg production is naturally stimulated by light and heat. Also beware of eggs that are "vegetarian fed." Chickens are natural omnivores and should be eating animal protein such as bugs and worms.

Simple Scrambled Eggs

A simple dish, but a little care in preparation will result in creamy soft curds rather than dry, rubbery pieces of eggs.

> **2 eggs**
> **1 yolk (optional)**
> **2 tablespoons fat or more (ghee, butter, bacon, duck, coconut oil)**
> **2 tablespoons cream (optional)**
> **Salt and pepper to taste**

1. Beat eggs, extra yolk, and cream well in a small bowl.

2. Heat fat over low to medium heat. Add egg mixture and keep stirring until soft curds start to appear (about 8 minutes). Cooking at a lower heat will take a few minutes longer, but the results will be softer and more creamy eggs. Lower heat also helps to retain the nutrients and enzymes.

Hard-Boiled Eggs

The easiest snack ever! Don't forget to also pack a bit of salt. One drawback of fresh eggs is that they are more challenging to shell when hard-boiled. In fresh eggs, the albumen (egg white) tends to stick to the inner shell membrane due to the less acidic environment of the egg.

After the eggshell's protective coat slowly wears off, the egg becomes porous, absorbs more air, and releases some of its carbon dioxide. This makes the albumen more acidic, causing it to stick to the inner membrane less. The egg white also shrinks slightly, so the air space between the eggshell and the membrane grows larger, resulting in boiled eggs that are easier to peel.

Two options for easy to peel fresh eggs—wait a week or add a teaspoon of baking soda to the water when boiling.

3 medium sized eggs
1 quart or more filtered water
1 teaspoon baking soda (optional for super fresh eggs)

1. Place eggs in small pot and cover with water with a least 1 inch of water over the eggs. Add a teaspoon of baking soda for super fresh eggs.

2. Bring eggs to a boil and than cover and turn off heat. Let eggs sit for at least 10 minutes or longer. Rinse in cool water and peel when ready to eat.

Cultured Egg Salad

4 hard-boiled eggs diced
1 scallion chopped
1 teaspoon fresh parsley hopped
Salt and pepper to taste
Dash smoked paprika
1 teaspoon nutritional yeast (optional but yummy)
1/4 teaspoon ground garlic powder or less fresh garlic
1/4 cup fermented mayonnaise
1 to 2 tablespoons sour cream

1. Place eggs and rest of ingredients in medium mixing bowl. Combine and adjust seasonings. Place in fridge for at least 30 minutes for flavors to set.

2. Serve with almost anything! Slices of cucumber/tomato, buckwheat crackers, nori seaweed wrap, lettuce wrap, or celery sticks.

Variations: Replace 1/2 of eggs with chopped boiled chicken, salmon or sardines. All are great options!

Crustless Quiche

I have so much fun making these since I can make several variations from one batch. They are good served warm or cold. After making them many times, I discovered a few tips and tricks that I can now share with you. A little tapioca starch gives this dish more of a smooth custard texture. And using muffin bake ware or small ramekins allows you to make several different types at once.

Most recipes call for "add-ins" like cheese, veggies, or chopped meat to the batter. I find that adding these ingredients in layers is a much more effective way to distribute *goodies* evenly.

> **6 to 7 eggs**
> **1/4 cup whole milk**
> **2.5 cups add-ins (chopped broccoli/mushrooms/scallions, bacon, chopped ham cubes)**
> **2 to 3 tablespoons butter (ghee, lard, bacon fat, coconut oil)**
> **2 teaspoons gluten free tamari or teaspoon Red Boat fish sauce**
> **3/4 cup shredded cheese (cheddar, Gruyere, Swiss) or small cubed pieces**
> **2 tablespoons chopped parsley/cilantro (optional)**
> **1/2 teaspoon salt**
> **1/2 teaspoon pepper**
> **1 tablespoon tapioca starch (optional)**

1. Preheat oven to 350°F.

2. In a large pan, saute add-ins. Be sure to chop add-ons into small pieces. Set aside.

3. In a large mixing bowl, combine eggs, tapioca starch, herbs, salt, pepper, tamari and milk.

4. Use butter or fat of choice to prepare muffin pan, ramekins or large quiche dish.

5. Evenly scatter chopped veggies/chopped bacon/ham into each muffin cup. Repeat with cheese.

6. Pour batter into each cup without overfilling (leave room for expansion). Push fork into each to be sure ingredients are at bottom and air pockets are reduced.

7. Bake for 35 minutes or until light brown on top. Do not overcook—they will continue to cook even after you remove them from the oven. Let cool for 15 to 20 minutes and then serve!

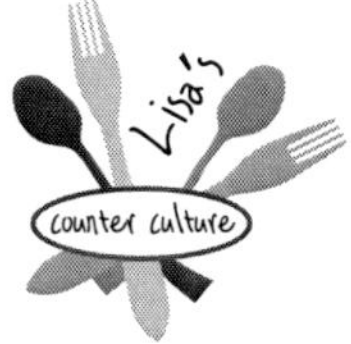

Organ Meat

While muscle meat offers plenty of protein, some wholesome fat, and a decent profile of micronutrients, it's the organ meat that represents the truly best source of many vitamins and minerals. Liver is one of the most nutrient-dense foods available: a 100-gram portion of lamb liver has more than twice the amount of folate and more than two-and-half times the amount vitamin A as a 100-gram portion of raw spinach. Organ meat is a vital food, brimming with nutrients.

Adding a small amount of liver or other organ meat into your diet, once or twice a week, can have a great impact on your intake of vitamins and minerals, particularly folate and vitamin A, which are critical to reproductive function and proper fetal development.

Traditionally, nose-to-tail eating was the norm; no part of the animal was left unused or wasted. Bones became mineral and collagen-rich broth and muscle meat was consumed. But organ meats were treasured, often saved for babies, nursing mothers, and the elderly.

From the Weston Price Website: Why Organ Meats?

> *Compared with muscle meats, organ meats are richer in just about every nutrient, including minerals like phosphorus, iron, copper, magnesium and iodine, and in B vitamins including B1, B2, B6, folic acid and especially vitamin B12. Organ meats provide high levels of the all-important fat-soluble vitamins A, D, E and K, especially if the animals live outside in the sunlight and eat green grass. Organ meats are also rich in beneficial fatty acids such as arachidonic acid, EPA and DHA. Organ meats even contain vitamin C—liver is richer in vitamin C than apples or carrots! Even if you add only small amounts of organ meats to your ground meat dishes, you are providing your family with super nutrition in ways that everyone likes and are easy to consume.*

I found the following compelling data on Tierra Soul's website. According to her post,

You will derive more nutrition from eating LIVER once a month than if you eat red meat every day. *Check out a comparison of nutrients in equal serving sizes of Liver and Steak. Liver is clearly superior to steak, but it is insane to think carrots or spinach could possibly compete in anything except the Calcium department.*

	Liver	**Steak**	**Carrots**	**Spinach**
Vitamin A	30485.26 IU	0.00 IU	34317.40 **	18865.80 IU
Vitamin B-12	41.39 mcg	2.92 mcg	0.00 mcg	0.00 mcg
Vitamin C	35.16 mg	0.00 mg	11.35 mg	17.64 mg
Vitamin D	13.61 IU	13.61 IU	0.00 mcg	-- IU
Folate	860.70 mcg	7.93 mcg	17.08 mcg	262.80 mcg
Vitamin E	0.57 IU	0.33 IU	0.84 IU	5.58 IU
Calcium	7.93 mg	7.93 mg	32.94 mg	244.80 mg
Iron	2.97 mg	4.05 mg	0.61 mg	6.43 mg
Magnesium	21.55 mg	34.03 mg	18.30 mg	156.60 mg

****Carrots: IU in the form of carotenes (which isn't really the same as Vitamin A)**

Ready. Set. Go!

Here is a collection of my easiest and quickest ways to prepare some of my family's favorite organ meats. Funny how kids who are raised eating these nutrient-dense foods can appreciate them first for how delicious they are and then later for how nutrient dense they are. It's important to give your taste buds a chance to get familiar with these new flavors and textures if they are new to you. I hope you will find these preparations as delicious as we do!

Chicken Liver Pate

It's funny how my kids will eat this dish almost nonstop. Once, they insisted on eating it for breakfast and lunch—all week long.

Note: The key to making this dish a hit with hesitant eaters is the ratio of thirds. Try to balance the ratio of chicken liver to eggs to onion/mushroom/garlic/seasonings to a third each. Also, be sure to let this chill overnight for the flavors to set.

6 to 8 servings

1/2 pound organic chicken liver
1 slice nitrate-free bacon (optional)
1/2 onion diced
Handful brown or oyster mushrooms sliced (optional but adds umami)
3 cloves garlic minced
Salt (at least 1 teaspoon probably more, tastes better when properly salted)
White pepper to taste
3 tablespoons fresh parsley minced
Dash cooking sherry or white wine or apple cider vinegar in a pinch
Organic pastured pork lard (or combo butter and lard or coconut oil, or bacon fat)
2 to 3 hard-boiled medium eggs

1. Rinse chicken livers gently.

2. Sauté 1/2 onion diced generous spoon of pork lard until onions are brownish and mushrooms are fully cooked if using. This concentrates the intensity of these flavors.

3. Set aside in a bowl to cool

4. Peel cooled hard-boiled eggs and set aside

5. Sauté remaining ingredients with pork lard/butter too but be sure to leave chicken livers a little pink—don't overcook!

6. Wait until all ingredients cool a bit—this is important so that it doesn't become total mushy glue when blending.

7. Add onion/mushroom mixture to food processor. Blend well.

8. Add eggs to food processor—pulse several times.

9. Add rest of mixture from the pan (chicken liver, garlic, parsley)

10. Pulse several seconds—taste—adjust salt/pepper. Try a dash of cumin. Chill before serving.

Serving Suggestion: Many people prefer to eat this spread on toast, fresh bread, or crackers. Gluten or grain-free alternatives include tomato slices, cucumber slices, celery stalks, or fresh greens as a wrap (arugula, spinach, endive).

Lamb Hearts

This recipe also works well with chicken hearts—of course you need many more per serving—at least 10 chicken hearts (or 20 if you ask my daughter,) per serving.

1 to 2 servings

> **One to two lamb hearts (one per person)**
> **Onion powder**
> **Clove garlic**
> **Salt and pepper to taste**
> **Lard (or coconut oil/ghee/bacon fat)**
> **Dash sherry or balsamic vinegar or plain kombucha**

1. Cut heart in half—discard fat or white pieces, Cut into ½ inch strips. Rinse and pat dry.

2. Heat lard in pan; add heart, seasonings and sherry Quickly sauté the heart keeping the pieces moving in the pan. Brown a bit—about 6 to 7 minutes at most. Don't overcook otherwise the texture gets rubbery.

Chicken Heart Variation: Cut many chicken hearts in 1/2—rinse and pat dry. At least 1/2 pound for two servings—there are really small.

Grill Variation: Cut trimmed lamb hearts into cubes and skewer for grill. Alternatively skewer whole chicken hearts and grill. Really tasty!

Note: If you have more time or want to get fancy, sauté some onions, mushrooms, and garlic before adding the heart. This is a similar process as the chicken liver pate. A nice addition when time permits. This doesn't often happen in my home.

Lamb Sweetbreads

A great way to introduce organ meat because of its mild and buttery flavor. This is also quicker and easier to prepare than beef sweetbreads which require a parboil first and than pressing.

1 to 2 servings

1 pound lamb sweetbreads
Organic lard/butter/coconut oil
Dash cumin
Salt and pepper to taste
Two cloves garlic minced
1 teaspoon onion powder (optional for browning instead of flour)
Splash sherry or brandy (optional)
1 tablespoon fresh parsley chopped or ½ teaspoon dry
Optional additions: mushrooms, onions, or scallions, jalapeño, parsley

1. Soak sweetbreads in cool filtered water for 30 minutes. Drain and rinse several times until the water is clear.

2. Separate into even bite-sized pieces either by pulling apart with hands or using a knife.

3. Remove more obvious fat pieces (see note). Pat dry.

4. Heat lard/butter/oil in pan. Add optional additions if using.

5. Sauté for several minutes. Add sweetbreads and remaining ingredients.

6. Sprinkle onion powder if using. This gives it the texture of being floured and nicely browns them.

7. Sauté until liquid evaporates and pieces start to brown. About 10 minutes or more.

8. Turn heat down and taste. If piece has light pink/white inside—they are ready to eat. These are not as sensitive to overcooking as the heart and liver.

Note: Most recipes have you discard the fat bits and remove any membrane. I find this time-consuming, and it doesn't really improve the finished dish. I do cook the little fat pieces along with the sweetbreads and scoop them out before the rest are done. They cook quickly and are a cook's treat.

Variation: Veal or young beef sweetbreads. Similar preparation and cooking. These are a bit larger lamb and may take a few minutes longer to cook. Cutting into smaller pieces decreases the cooking time. And for kids, they are ready to eat without you having to cut at the table!

Lamb or Goat Lengua (Tongue)

This recipe can also be used for beef tongue, which will take longer to cook. One beef tongue will make about 6 to 8 servings. Triple remaining ingredients for one beef tongue. The longer you cook it (9 hours or more), the more tender it will be.

2-3 servings

6 to 8 lamb/goat tongues (or 1 beef tongue for 6 to 8 servings)
1 onion cut in quarters
1 or 2 carrots
Celery stalk
Several garlic cloves
1 teaspoon each cumin/cinnamon/oregano
2 teaspoons salt and pepper
¼ cup filtered water or broth

1. Add all ingredients to slow cooker—Set on high for two to three hours or low for four or five hours.

2. Check to see if the tongue is tender by piercing it with a fork…the membrane should be loose and easy to remove. Discard membrane.

3. Shred tongue with fork or fingers into mixing/serving bowl

4. Add some parsley, oregano, sea salt, pepper—a bit of cayenne if you want a little heat.

5. Add a little of the broth.

6. Mix and taste. Adjust seasonings.

Serving Suggestions

- Eat as is.
- Add taco add-ons such as salsa, tomatillo salsa, guacamole, and sour cream. Wrap in corn tortillas or romaine leaves.
- Serve over rice with beans.

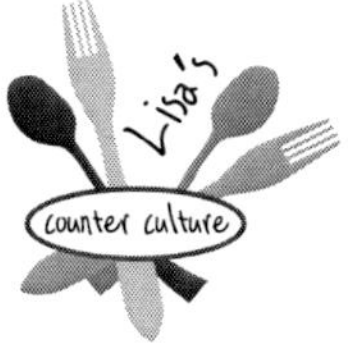

Seafood

I love seafood! I especially love anything with a shell and fish roe. Lucky me since they are some of the more nutrient-dense options available.

Choosing Seafood

Local, sustainable, and wild seafood will usually provide you with the freshest and tastiest options. However, other factors are also important. Smaller fish/shellfish are lower in problematic toxins such as mercury than the larger species since there are at the bottom of the food chain. Mollusks (Oysters, mussels, cockles and clams) are great particularly great options since you are consuming the whole animal, organs and all.

I prefer to choose seafood that already has a lot of flavor, so I don't have to spend time on fancy sauces and more intricate preparation. This means "fatty" fish like salmon, sardines, mackerel and sablefish. I like to be able to grill or broil with a bit of salt, pepper and lemon and dig in!

For sustainable options, be sure to check the Monterey Bay Aquarium **website** for the current recommendations of sustainable options in order to avoid supporting over-fishing.

I believe the benefits of eating fish outweigh the risks if you choose your fish carefully.

True Crab Cakes

Adapted from Mark Bittman, *The Minimalist* series.
4 servings

These are amazing, practically grain-free, and gluten-free. You can leave out the final dusting of brown rice flour. Make extra for snacks since they keep well.

The key step to making these amazing crab cakes—which actually taste like crab—is the pureed shrimp, which acts like glue to hold these cakes together. So there's no need for bread crumbs!

6 medium raw shrimp, shelled, washed and deveined (or 1/4 pound scallops)
1 teaspoon Red Boat fish sauce
1 pound fresh lump crab meat, picked over for cartilage
1 egg
1/4 cup chopped scallion
1/4 cup chopped cilantro
1/2 teaspoon fresh chili, preferably Thai, minced (remove seeds)
1 teaspoon minced fresh ginger
Salt and freshly ground black pepper
Coconut oil or ghee
1/2 cup brown rice flour (optional: great for crisp crust and browning)
Lime wedges for serving

1. Purée shrimp, fish sauce, garlic, chili and ginger in a food processor (smaller is better) until you have a smooth paste, or chop and mash by hand.

2. In a bowl, mix the purée, crab meat, egg, scallion, cilantro, salt and pepper.

3. Refrigerate mixture until you are ready to cook. It is easier to shape into cakes if you refrigerate it for 30 minutes or more.

4. Film bottom of a large skillet with oil and place over medium-high heat. Shape crab meat mixture into cakes 1-inch thick and as wide as you want.

5. Dredge each in brown rice flour, and cook, adjusting heat as necessary. Turn once (very gently), until golden brown on both sides, about 5 minutes a side. Serve with lime wedges.

Braised Squid with Artichokes

Adapted from Mark Bittman, *New York Times* Food Section.
3 to 4 servings

The anchovy/fish sauce really makes this dish sing. There's a great video to see a quick lesson on making these at dinersjournal.blogs.nytimes.com/2012/04/09/the-minimalist-braised-squid-with-artichokes/

2 medium artichokes, trimmed , fuzzy center near heart removed and halved
3 tablespoons coconut oil or ghee or lard (add olive oil before serving)
3 large cloves or more of minced garlic
1.5 to 2 ounces Red Boat fish sauce (or 2 anchovy fillets chopped)
2 pounds cleaned squid, the bodies cut into rings—these shrink so if you
  have big eaters—get an extra pound
1/8 cup white wine or cooking sherry, kombucha
Freshly ground black pepper
Minced parsley for garnish

1. Place a large saucepan or pot over medium heat and add 2 tablespoons of the oil. A minute later, add the garlic and fish sauce. Cook, stirring occasionally, until the anchovies break up and the garlic begins to color, 1 to 2 minutes. Add the squid, artichokes and wine. Stir, cover, and turn heat to medium.

2. The squid releases a **lot** of juice so you can serve this as a stew or drain some of the broth before serving.

3. Uncover and stir the mixture every 5 minutes or so.

4. When the squid and artichokes begin to become tender, after 15 or 20 minutes, uncover and cook until most of the liquid has evaporated and the squid and artichokes are tender, about 10 to 15 minutes longer.

5. Season with pepper. It's highly unlikely this dish will need added salt, especially if you use fish sauce/anchovies, but taste and see.

6. Stir in the remaining olive oil, garnish with the parsley and serve.

Salmon Goat Cheese Roll-Ups

This makes a great satisfying snack and is a big favorite with my kids. I often pack these for school lunches.

Wild smoked salmon
Chevre style goat cheese or kefir/yogurt cheese
Toasted nori sheets

1. Lay out seaweed flat. If using larger sheets, I usually cut in ½ to get it to fit into the lunch box sushi holder—smear some cheese on two-inch wide strip.

2. Add a slice of smoke salmon

3. Roll and eat!

Variations

- Replace smoked salmon with cooked salmon (leftovers are great for this)
- Replace smoked salmon with salmon roe (Ikura). This is a huge favorite with my kids.
- Try tuna and fermented mayonnaise.
- Salmon sashimi chopped with spicy mayonnaise.
- Add additional items such as cilantro, parsley, avocado and/or rice.

Steamed Shellfish

Just takes about 15 minutes! (This is the same recipe as the Cheater Fish Stock.)

1 to 2 pounds of cleaned mussels, clams or cockles in the shell
Filtered water
Dash sherry (optional)
Salt, pepper and spices (parsley, cilantro and/or lemongrass)
Clove garlic crushed
Butter pat or dash olive oil for serving

1. Place all ingredients in a small stock pot, add water to cover. Turn heat to high and close lid.

2. Shake occasionally to stir up the pot. Shellfish should start to open in 3 to 5 minutes—clams take longer and, in general, larger shells take longer than smaller ones.

3. As soon as all the shells open, they are ready to serve.

Optional: Add a tablespoon or two of butter/olive oil to serving bowl. This is also great with a bit of coconut milk and a pinch of saffron.

Broiled or Grilled Fish

Serves 4

I like fish that has lots of flavor and fat, so I don't have to do much cooking to enjoy it. The key is getting super fresh, high quality fish. Wild salmon, butterfish (aka sablefish), and sardines are my top picks. Any smaller oily fish are generally good choices in that they are lower in mercury and other toxins, since they are further down on the food chain. And the healthy, important long-chain omega-3 fatty acids EPA and DHA are very bioavailable. These fish are also high in selenium, which is good protection against mercury toxicity.

1 to 1.5 pounds fish steaks or fillets or for whole cleaned sardines
Salt and pepper to taste
Garlic powder or paste spread
Lemon slices for serving
Fermented garlic mayonnaise for serving (optional)

Using the broiler

1. Clean fish and pat dry. Lightly season with salt, pepper and garlic if desired.

2. Place fish on broiler rack/pan about 4 inches below the broiler element.

3. Broil for 3 to 5 minutes depending on thickness of fish. Note that the fish will keep cooking after you remove it, so don't overdo it. Be sure to flip fish if using a steaks cut.

4. For **sardines**, salt and pepper inside of fish, add some herbs and lemon slices if desired. Follow steps 1 through 3 above.

Using the grill

1. Clean fish and pat dry. Lightly season with salt, pepper and garlic if desired.

2. Place fish on medium hot grill.

3. Grill for 3 to 5 minutes depending on thickness of fish. Note that the fish will keep cooking after you remove it, so don't overdo it. Be sure to flip fish if using a steaks cut.

4. For **sardines**, salt and pepper inside of fish, add some herbs and lemon slices if desired. Follow steps 1 through 3 above.

Shrimp and Chive Dumplings

Step up and have some dim sum! Even without the traditional wrapper, these little gems are a winner! I was very surprised how toothsome and satisfying I found them.

Serves 4

1 pound raw shrimp peeled (reserve shells for a quick broth, page 78)
1/4 cup chopped garlic chives
Pinch of salt and pepper
1 tablespoon chopped cilantro (optional)
Gluten-free tamari, coconut aminos or garlic mayonnaise for dipping

1. Blend 1/2 peeled shrimp, salt, pepper and cilantro until it's almost a paste.

2. Add remaining shrimp and chives and pulse to pieces. Don't worry if you over process a little. They still come out great.

3. Roll a small bowl of the mixture with your hands (wet hands make it less sticky on your hands). The dumplings expand as they cook, so keep the balls on the small size.

4. Place the mixture balls on a parchment-lined steamer, insert over water. Steam until cooked through, about 8 to 10 minutes.

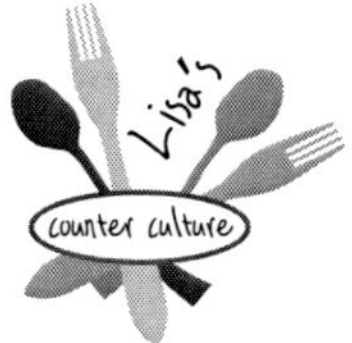

Meat

Protein is essential for normal growth, hormones, blood clotting and for lactation for feeding our babies. Animal protein is our only source of complete protein. Our early ancestors subsisted on a diet comprised mostly of meat and fat with some vegetables, fruit, nuts and seeds. Usable vitamin B12 occurs only in animal products. Animal fats supply vitamins A and D, which are necessary for assimilating proteins.

However, much negative press and health conditions have been associated with poor quality meat. It is important to source your meat as much as possible from properly raised livestock. Beef, lamb and goat should all be grassfed and pastured with no antibiotics or growth hormones. Similarly, chicken and pork should be pastured-raised and not fed a diet of GMO soy and corn.

High quality meat retains more nutrients and flavor when serving it rare, braised or slow roasted at lower heat. Try to avoid high heat preparations to avoid elevated carcinogens. Avoid processed meats such as bacon, sausage, luncheon meat preserved with nitrates and other meat preservatives. Traditional cultures used lactofermentation, salt curing or smoking to prepare these products.

Most people who recommend "lean meat" are assuming that you only have access to conventionally-farmed, grain-fed meat. Grain-fed meat has an unfavorable omega-6:omega-3 ratio. Where grass-fed fat shines and grain-fed fat fails is in the anti-carcinogenic conjugated linoleic acid (CLA) content, which is far higher in grassfed meat and fat. CLA is a fatty acid that has recently been studied as a potent cancer fighter.

That said, it's better to eat lean conventional meat rather than none at all. If all you can afford or have access to is grain-fed meat, trim the excess fat, and counter the leanness by incorporating a nice fat-based sauce.

Did you know?

- Meat from grass-fed animals has two to four times more omega-3 fatty acids than meat from grain-fed animals.
- When chickens are kept indoors and deprived of greens, their meat and eggs also become artificially low in omega-3s.
- The meat from the pastured cattle is four times higher in vitamin E than the meat from the feedlot.

Pastured pork can be a wondrous protein. It packs a lot of flavor! One trick I have found in making burgers with grassfed beef is to add either a slice or two of chopped bacon or 20% by weight of ground pork to the mixture. Grassfed ground can be a little too lean for great burgers, depending on the ground mixture you are using. And of course, there is lard! A great stable fat for sauteing or frying without oxidizing!

What to do with leftover chicken

- Chicken/Egg Salad (fermented mayonnaise, chopped chicken, hard-boiled egg, cilantro, chopped pickle, ground pepper and salt)
- Chicken Veggie Stew (broth, chopped chicken, chopped veggies, garlic and onion)
- Chicken Casserole (layered refried beans, cheese, salsa, chicken, fresh corn/ cooked zucchini)

Using bacon

Besides just eating cooked strips of uncured pastured bacon, there are a few more favorites I would like to share.

- Chop half a slice into small bits and saute in a pan that you are about use to make scrambled eggs. A little bit cooks up quick and lends a lot flavor and good fats.
- Chop and add to burgers.
- Take several slices and drape over the top of meatloaf to keep it moist and amazing.
- Make almost any vegetable way better. I have found that roasting chopped bacon with Brussels sprouts has converted many a sprout hater to lover.
- Save the bacon drippings! A wonderful way to saute eggs or vegetables or warm to add to salad dressings. Don't waste this heat-stable nutrient rich fat!

Slow Cooker Chicken

It's amazingly easy and tender. You won't need a knife to carve this one! If your slow cooker is large enough, cook two chickens and use the leftovers for lunch!

> **3 to 4 pound whole chicken**
> **1 large onion coarsely chopped**
> **2 teaspoons salt**
> **2 teaspoon paprika**
> **1 teaspoon onion powder**
> **1 teaspoon garlic powder**
> **1 teaspoon ground pepper**
> **2 teaspoons oregano**

1. Wash and dry chicken (be sure to remove neck and giblets if needed)

2. Place chopped onions on bottom of slow cooker.

3. Combine spices in a small bowl. Run spice mixture over chicken and even under the skin.

4. Place chicken breast side up in slow cooker. No liquid is needed. The chicken will make the gravy over the onions as they caramelize.

5. Cover and turn on high. Cook for 4 to 5 hours. Baste if you want.

Foolproof Baby Back Ribs

Serves 4

The key here is "slow and low" to get extra tender, fall off the bones ribs. I skip seasoning or basting while cooking. These taste wonderful as is, but you can add salt/sauce if desired.

> **2 racks or about 5 pounds baby back ribs**
> **Salt and pepper to taste**
> **BBQ sauce (optional)**

1. Preheat oven to 275°F.

2. Cut racks in 1/2 so that they easily fit onto a baking sheet. Place back-side up. (Optional: remove the thin membrane on the back side of the ribs. Also easy to do this after it's done cooking.)

3. Turn every 30 minutes for at least 2 hours total. If you cook for an additional hour or two at a lower heat (225°F) and flip ribs a few more times, then the meat will be even more tender.

4. That's it! Remove and serve!

Super Easy Carnitas

Use Large Slow Cooker (Crock Pot)

A few minutes of preparation in the morning, and by dinner, you will have a great meal! Make extra; the leftovers taste even better the next day.

A fermented apple cider really makes the recipe stand out with very tender and flavorful results. I've used stout or beer, but I haven't found one that is gluten free. Alternatively, you could use chicken broth.

> **1 (3 to 4 pounds) boneless pork shoulder roast**
> **4 to 6 garlic cloves or more**
> **1 teaspoon ground cumin**
> **1/2 teaspoon crumbled dried oregano**
> **1/2 teaspoon ground coriander**
> **1/4 teaspoon ground cinnamon**
> **1 teaspoon salt**
> **2 cups fermented cider or gluten free beer**
> **One onion chopped**

1. Mix together in a bowl salt, garlic powder, cumin, oregano, coriander, and cinnamon. Coat pork with the spice mixture. You can leave the pork butt whole, but I usually cut it into four pieces to cook a bit quicker.

2. Place pork and onions into cooker. Pour the cider or broth around the sides of the pork, being careful not to rinse off the spice mixture.

3. Cover and cook on high for 1 hour and then set to low for the rest of the time (8 hours or so) until the pork shreds easily with a fork.

4. Turn the meat after it has cooked for 4 hours.

5. When the pork is tender, remove from slow cooker, and shred with two forks. Use cooking liquid as needed to moisten the meat. Adjust salt and pepper and be sure to fish out garlic cloves to mash into the meat.

Mini Patties

This is a dish that my grandmother made for me when I was growing up. I never got her exact recipe. She often used ground turkey or chicken thigh, but I prefer to use ground pork for the higher fat content and flavor. I think I captured the essence of my grandmother's recipe, and it is an often requested dish in my home.

Makes 10 patties

1 pound ground meat (1/2 veal and 1/2 pork)
1 medium egg beaten (duck eggs are great for holding the patties together)
1 small onion chopped fine
3 cloves garlic minced
1 teaspoon Red Boat fish sauce
Two small tomatoes pureed
Handful mushrooms chopped fine
2 tablespoons fresh parsley chopped
1 teaspoon salt and white pepper
2 tablespoons lard, ghee or bacon fat

1. Saute lard, onions and mushrooms until soft. Add garlic and stir. After one minute, remove from heat. Cool five minutes.

2. In a large bowl, mix egg, fish sauce, tomato, parsley and spices. Mix in ground meat and cooled mixture from pan and combine gently. Don't overwork the meat.

3. Form into small 4-inch patties. Broil or sauté in pan for 3 minutes each side. Variation: Bake at 350°F for 15 to 20 minutes.

4. Serve warm or cold. Tastes even better the next day.

The Best Meatloaf Ever

Based on a recipe from Fine Cooking. The key is bacon! A few strips over the top of the loaf while baking makes this dish stand out! It also keeps the loaf moist. Never serve dry meatloaf again!

1.5 pounds ground meat (mix of beef, veal and pork)
4 strips bacon
2 eggs beaten (duck eggs are great since they hold things together)
1.5 teaspoons Red Boat fish sauce or two chopped anchovies (optional)
1/4 cup fresh parsley chopped
1/2 teaspoon ground mustard or 1 teaspoon prepared mustard
2 large tomatoes pureed
1 onion chopped fine
3 to 4 cloves garlic minced
1.5 teaspoons salt
3/4 teaspoon ground pepper
1 tablespoon lard, ghee or bacon fat

1. Heat oven to 350°F. In small skillet, heat the lard, add onions and cook over medium heat until soft—about 4 minutes.

2. Add garlic and saute another 1 to 2 minutes. Set aside to cool.

3. In a large mixing bowl, combine all the remaining ingredients—except the bacon—and add the cooled onion-garlic mixture. Mix with a rubber spatula or your hands just until the ingredients are combined. Don't overwork the meat.

4. Oil a rimmed baking sheet or a large casserole dish. Turn the meat mixture out onto the pan and shape it into a large loaf.

5. Wrap strips of bacon around the shaped loaf, tucking the ends under the loaf.

6. Bake the meatloaf until an instant-read thermometer registers 160°F, 50 to 60 minutes for a large loaf. Before slicing, let the meatloaf rest for 10 to 15 minutes to allow some carryover cooking and to let the juices redistribute. To serve, slice and spoon some of the pan juices over the slices, if you like.

Quick Steaks (Grill or Broil)

Grassfed steaks (grassfed and grass-finished) taste best medium rare; otherwise, they tend to taste like leather. A few adjustments and you will end up with great tasting steaks. Grassfed also tends to be leaner, which makes it more challenging to keep tender. A little marbling goes a long way for flavor and a buttery mouth feel while chewing. Grassfed meat cooks quicker, since it retains less water than its bloated grain-fed counterparts.

Here are my top three go-to favorite cuts, ranked by cost:

Least Expensive. Tri-tip is trickier to prepare as one large piece of meat. The smaller pointed ends cook faster than the middle. (We prefer medium rare, which is not doable with a whole piece.) One big piece takes much longer to cook. Steaks are the way to go!

Mid-Range Price. Skirt steak is our favorite. It has nice marbling, so you end up with a very tender piece of meat. These steaks are usually thin cut, so they are quick to cook. Flank steak is great for cutting up for fajitas, too.

Most Expensive. Boneless ribeye. This is a special occasion steak in our house.

Tips

- Bring meat to room room temperature, at least 30 to 45 minutes before cooking (longer if your home is cold).
- Grassfed meat is quite lean and is best with a fat-based marinade. Unfiltered extra virgin olive oil has enzymes that tenderize and keep the meat moist.
- Avoid using vinegar, wine or acids in marinades for grassfed meat as they will make the meat tough.
- For even cooking, be sure all the steaks are the same thickness. When cutting the Tri-tip into steaks—1 inch is great. Flatten if necessary to make even.
- Smaller pieces cook faster than larger pieces. I usually cut the Tri-tip into 6 to 8 inch long pieces before grilling.
- Grassfed steaks are lean, so they taste best medium-rare (internal temp 125°F); otherwise, they tend to get tough when cooked longer.
- Boneless meat cooks much faster than bone-in.
- When grilling or broiling, let meat rest for 10 minutes after cooking to keep it moist and juicy.

Using the grill

An indirect heat source is ideal. For example, if you have a three burner grill, then:

1. Turn on all three to high for several minutes.

2. Turn off middle burner and place meat over this area of the grill. Close lid.

3. Skirt steak cooks the quickest (about 3 to 4 minutes a side).

4. Let rest for 10 minutes after removing from heat to keep your steaks moist and juicy.

Using the broiler

1. Turn broiler on. Wait a few minutes and then set steaks on flat pan with lip about 4 to 5 inches below the element.

2. Broil for 2 to 3 minutes each side (internal temp of 125°F)

3. Let meat rest for 8 to 10 minutes before serving.

Asian Slow-Cooker Short Ribs

Serves 4

This is a super easy "fix it and forget it" recipe. You can get fancy and brown the ribs first, but I never bother. (Who needs more dishes to clean, and I don't taste a big difference.)

> **4 to 5 pounds bone-in English-style grass-fed short ribs**
> **2 tablespoons Red Boat fish sauce**
> **1/2 cup gluten-free tamari or coconut aminos**
> **1 cup broth (beef or chicken)**
> **6 to 8 cloves garlic**
> **2 inches peeled chopped fresh ginger**
> **1/2 teaspoon salt and pepper**
> **Medium tart apple**
> **3 to 4 scallions chopped or small onion chopped**

1. Place the ribs into a slow cooker, so they are in one layer if possible.

2. Puree remaining ingredients until smooth to make the sauce.

3. Pour sauce over the ribs.

4. Cook for 5 to 6 hours (until meat falls off the bone).

5. Turn off heat and let meat rest for 15 minutes before serving.

Stir-Fry Chicken

This is a quick dish, once you have prepped the veggies. Be sure to use fresh ginger.

> **1 teaspoon fresh minced ginger**
> **2 cloves garlic minced**
> **Large handful mushrooms sliced (Shitake or Crimini)**
> **4 scallions chopped**
> **1 red bell pepper chopped**
> **1/2 pound snap peas or sugar snap peas**
> **1/2 pound bok choy quartered or other green vegetable**
> **2 tablespoons gluten free tamari**
> **1.5 teaspoons tapioca starch (optional—acts as thickener)**
> **3/4 pound boneless skinless chicken sliced into strips**
> **3 tablespoons coconut oil, lard or ghee**

1. In a large skillet or wok, set at medium heat, stir-fry half of coconut oil and mushrooms until well cooked. Add chicken, 1 tablespoon tamari, and scallions.

2. Sprinkle tapioca starch over chicken if using. Stir-fry until chicken is no longer pink. Take care to not overcook. Remove and keep warm.

3. In the same pan, stir-fry the remaining oil, vegetables and seasonings for 3 to 4 minutes. Return chicken/mushrooms to the pan; mix well. Heat through and let juices thicken for a few minutes.

4. Taste, adjust seasonings, salt and pepper. Serve.

Variations: Replace chicken with shrimp, beef or pork. Replace chicken with cooked cubed chicken added towards end of cooking.

Sides

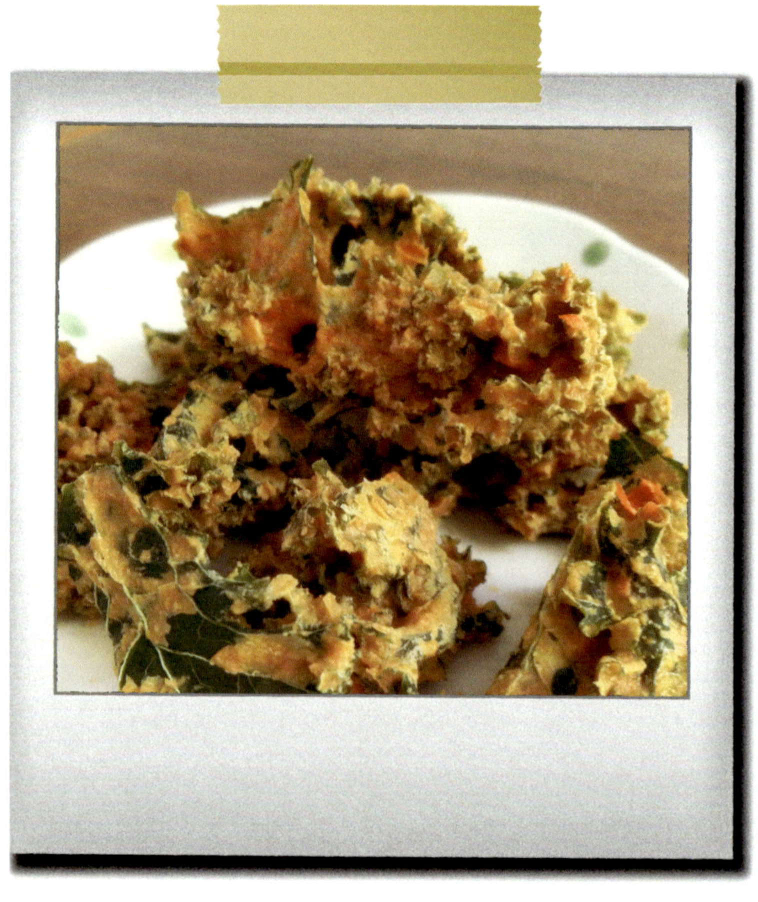

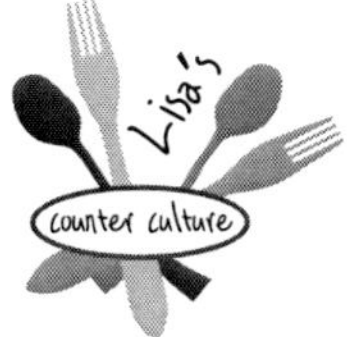

Sides

There are endless side dishes that you can serve with your meals. I usually offer both raw and cooked vegetables with each meal and a starch on occasion. Most of my side dishes are pretty obvious recipes—cutting up ingredients and roasting, steaming or sauteing. The few recipes that I share here are the ones that I think you may find most useful.

Pureed Greens

A very easy and digestible way to eat a variety of greens. This is my version of an Indian style dish.

> **One bunch greens or mixture (kale, chard, spinach, baby bok choy)**
> **1/2 onion chopped**
> **1/4 to 1/2 cup ghee, lard or coconut oil**
> **1 to 2 cloves garlic minced**
> **Cilantro/parsley (optional)**
> **Salt and pepper to taste**
> **Dash cumin, ginger, and cinnamon**

1. Add ghee, lard or coconut oil to pan on low heat.

2. Add chopped onions and saute until soft.

3. Add greens, herbs and spices and cook until quite soft.

4. Puree to your liking and adjust seasonings if needed.

Artichokes

This is a favorite vegetable in our home. Serve it with fermented mayonnaise and garlic. Delectable!

Artichokes are a simple vegetable to cook, but many people new to artichokes are scared by their appearance. Take a chance and try this recipe—it's super simple!

3 medium to small artichokes
Water
Salt

1. Cut the stem potion of the artichoke and discard. Trim the upper pointed leaves of the artichoke—this is usually the top 1/2 to 1 inch of the artichoke.

2. Place the artichokes stem side down in a sauce pan, and fit snugly.

3. Add water to 1/2 way up on the artichoke sides.

4. Cover with lid and bring to a boil.

5. Turn down to simmer and cook about 15 minutes or until stem part is easily pieced with a fork.

6. Drain and serve. Scrap the leaves from the stem section and than scrape out the fuzzies when you get to the "heart." Serve garlic mayonnaise for dipping.

Zucchini Noodles

I love using my spiral slicer! (See page 131). My favorite noodles are made from zucchini. A few minutes of prep, a few minutes of cooking, and you end up with great tasting noodles that are good for you!

Serves 4

2 to 3 large straight fresh zucchini (peeled has a similar texture to regular noodles)
1/2 teaspoon salt

1. Use very firm and straight summer squash to easily make glorious long noodles.

2. Cut two very straight edges on ends of zucchini. Place into the spiral slicer. Using the larger of the two noodle attachments and start turning! Put a plate or small bowl to catch the noodles coming out.

3. Lightly salt and toss. Set aside for 15 minutes. Use a towel or your hands to wring out any excess water. Heat large skillet or pot with fat of your choice and saute several minutes. Toss with sauce or serve as is.

About Rice

I recommend using white aromatic rice instead of brown rice. I know this seems to be the opposite of what most health professionals tell you. But I consider rice a "fun" or safer starch in that it does not have gluten and the aromatic (jasmine and basmati) have a lower glycemic index than brown.

From Mark's Daily Apple Blog:

The common thread is that white, milled, polished rice is basically pure starch. All the chemical negatives are found in the hull, husk, and bran, and those are easily removed or negated. It is essentially a blank slate, nothing all that bad about it, but nothing all that great, either.

Nutrient wise, there is not much difference between brown and white rice, and the negatives (phytates and arsenic, and more) are easily avoided with white. Rice can be a great vehicle for nutrient dense foods such as butter, coconut milk, and stews.

Coconut or Broth Rice

I like to rinse rice thoroughly and then let it sit for a few hours in fresh water. Drain, rinse again, and then cook. I find that this technique has less of an effect on my blood sugar.

Of course, serve this with a healthy fat and protein to offset the carbohydrate load. Feel free to double the recipe and use the extra rice throughout the week.

1 cup basmati or other aromatic rice
Coconut milk (or part water) to cover rice with 1 inch over rice
Pinch of saffron (optional but lends a beautiful color and subtle flavor)

1. Place drained rice (after rinsing and soaking) into pot. Cover with coconut milk/water to 1 inch over the rice surface)

2. Cover and bring to a low boil.

3. Turn heat down to simmer and cook until liquid is absorbed (about 15 minutes)

4. Fluff and serve. Season with salt if desired.

Broth rice variation: Replace coconut milk with bone broth.

Crunchy Nut Chutney

Adapted from Mark Bittman's *How To Cook Everything*. You may want to double this recipe because it's quite addictive.

Makes 1/2 cup

> **1/2 teaspoon cumin seeds**
> **1/2 teaspoon coriander seeds**
> **1/2 dried Thai or other small red chili, or more to taste**
> **1/2 cup roasted unsalted cashews (almonds, or other nut)**
> **1/4 teaspoon salt**
> **1/4 teaspoon freshly ground black pepper**
> **1/2 clove garlic or more, peeled**

1. Toast all seeds and chili in a small dry skillet over medium heat until the seeds color lightly—about 5 minutes.

2. Process all ingredients together in food processor, scraping down the sides as necessary. Taste, adjust seasoning, and serve at room temperature. Be careful not to make nut butter

Variation: Add dried fruit (raisins or dried cherries work well)

Note: Increase the digestibility of this dish by using crispy nuts as described in *Nourishing Traditions*.

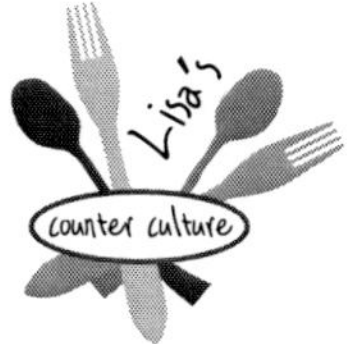

Dehydrator

I love using my Excalibur 9-Tray Dehydrator. It's so versatile. Besides the expected dried fruit and herbs. this is a great tool for making jerky, gluten free crackers, fruit or kefir leathers, veggie crackers, kale chips, crispy nuts and yogurt! You can even dehydrate bone broth!

I have included several of my favorite recipes in this section. But there are endless possibilities for using your dehydrator to make nutrient-dense foods and to preserve foods for enjoyment later in the season.

I have included two dehydrator recipes in this book. Additionally, you can get a great granola recipe on the Pickl-It website.

- Kefir Leather on page 54
- Raw Milk Yogurt on page 57

The Excalibur Dehydration Guide is full of great recipes and ideas and information on preserving the enzymes and nutrients in your food. According to the booklet, they found through testing samples for enzymatic content that temperatures up to 145°F was the same as food dried at lower temperature. There is a difference between the food temperature versus the air temperature during the dehydration process. Food temperatures tend to be about 20 to 30 °F lower the air temp due to the effects of evaporation.

You can even preserve the probiotic content of your kefir and yogurt leathers as well as other dehydrated veggies. Try making dehydrated pickles! Make your own seasoning powders, too. I love dehydrating shiitake mushrooms and then blending them into a powder for seasoning our meals.

Buckwheat Flax Crackers

These are surprisingly good for a "healthy" cracker. I've also made these with leftover veggie pulp from juicing instead of using flax seeds. You may want to double this recipe!

2 cups raw untoasted buckwheat groats
1/4 cup whole flaxseeds
1 large tomato or 2 medium tomatoes
1 red or yellow bell pepper
2 cloves garlic
1 teaspoon salt

1. Soak buckwheat groats overnight with filtered water and a tablespoon of lemon juice.

2. Place all ingredients in a high-speed blender or food processor. Blend until fine consistency is reached.

3. Spread mixture evenly on paraflex or parchment paper on a dehydrator sheet.

4. Gently score with a dull knife into squares.

5. Dehydrate at 135°F for 8 to 10 hours. Check after 4 hours to see if the crackers are solid.

6. Once the crackers are solid, remove from the sheets and place on the mesh sheets and continue until completely dry and crispy.

Dehydrated Bone Broth

Courtesy of Patty of Loving Our Guts at lovingourguts.com
Modified slightly.

Bone broth (unsalted) (any type)

1. Gently boil your broth to 1/3 of its original volume. Careful not to burn it.

2. After broth has thickened, you are ready to dehydrate.

3. Pour a thin layer onto a paraflex sheet.

4. Set at highest temperature. Drying time will be between 48 and 72 hours. Flip every 24 hours or so.

5. When broth no longer sticks to the sheets, you are ready to process it into a powder for storage. Or keep for broth leathers.

6. Powder can easily be used by adding hot water or sprinkled over hot veggies.

Almost Cheesy Kale Chips (Dairy Free)

My kids love these chips. They are so quick to make, and they cost a fraction of what the health food stores sell them. Try using different types of kale or even chard!

1 large bunch curly kale or dino kale
1/2 teaspoon salt
1 red bell pepper, seeded and chopped
1 cup cashews soaked for at least 2 hours in filtered water
Juice 1 lemon
2 tablespoons nutritional yeast

1. Take cleaned and dry kale and remove the large stems. Tear into large bite-sized pieces (kale will shrink while drying)

2. Blend red pepper, salt, drained cashews, lemon and nutritional yeast until smooth.

3. Be prepared to get messy! With clean hands and a large bowl, massage the mixture all over the kale.

4. Place kale pieces onto the screen sheets of the dehydrator. They don't need to lie flat.

5. Dehydrate at 115°F overnight or until coating is dry.

6. Flip and place onto mesh screens until crispy (a few more hours).

Jammin Jerky

I love this recipe since it doesn't have any nasty chemicals or preservatives. It's super easy and not too salty.

Jerky works best with very lean cuts of meat. Leaner cuts can be stored longer. Grassfed and/or pastured jerky is hard to find commercially and tends to be costly. Make it yourself and save a bundle!

1/2 cup apple cider vinegar
1/4 cup gluten free tamari or coconut aminos
Thinly sliced lean meat (beef, buffalo, lamb, venison)

1. Mix apple cider vinegar and tamari in a medium flat dish with sides. Choose something large enough to dunk meat pieces.

2. Slice meat into strips 4 to 5 inches long and 1 inch wide.

3. Dunk strips into mixture and lay flat onto the dehydrator sheets. This works well for me, but you could also try marinating it longer in the fridge for more flavor.

4. Dry at 155°F for 4 to 6 hours. Blot any fat droplets that appear on the surface. You can also skip this part—I often forget to do it, and it still turns out great.

5. Always test a cooled piece. The jerky should be able to bend/crack without breaking.

6. Store in airtight containers or vacuum-sealed bags. Keep in dark cool place for best results.

Treats

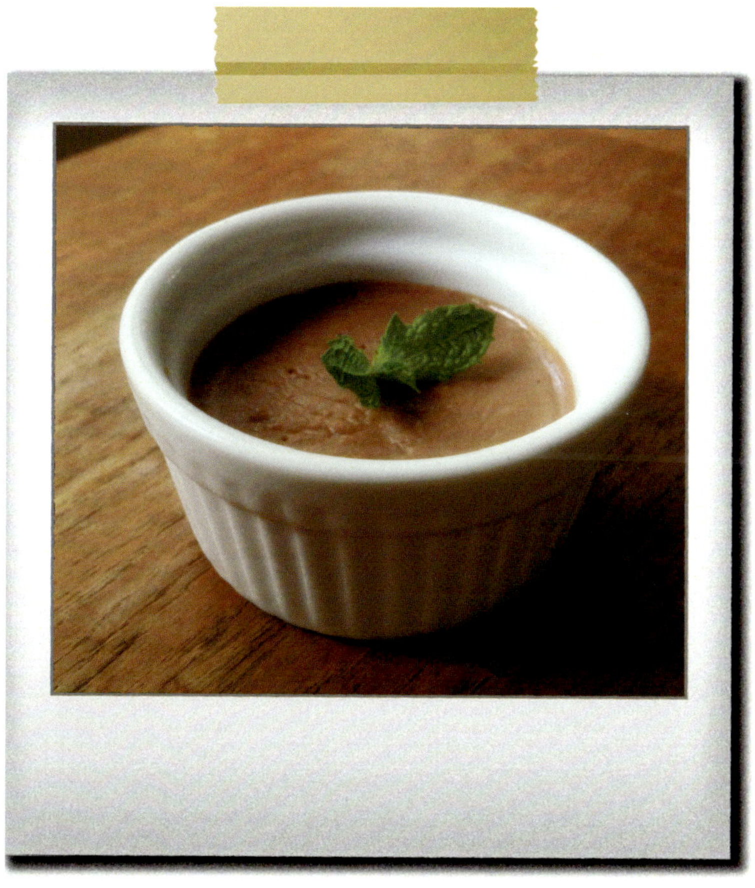

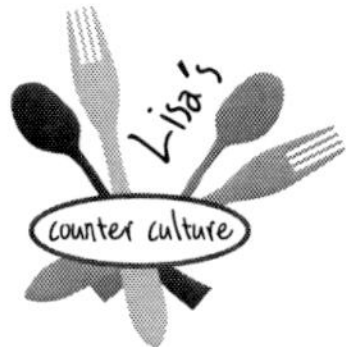

Treats

Treats can be a great way to sneak in nutrient dense foods while feeling indulged. High quality ingredients and attention to portions can make treats a worthy part of your diet.

I feel that treats should taste great, and a little can go a long way. When my family goes out, I often see people are surprised when we share one small dessert like a custard, rather than each one of us having our own. My children, husband and I will all take turns enjoying small bites and savoring them as we go. I like to choose treats that are not just sugar bombs, but that are balanced with healthy fat and some nutrients, too.

I've listed a few of the regular desserts on our rotation. I also scattered a few recipes earlier in the book (fruit leathers, kefir ice cream and smoothies).

Dairy-Free Soft Serve Ice Cream

Serves 2 (or in my house, 4)

> **2 frozen sliced bananas (freeze after slicing)**
> **2 tablespoons almond butter**
> **1-2 tablespoons raw honey**
> **1 tablespoon organic cocoa powder or dark chocolate ground**
> **1/2 teaspoon vanilla**

1. Combine all ingredients in a food processor. Process for 5 minutes until creamy.

2. Variations: Substitute 1/2 cup pureed fruit (apricot, peaches, etc.) and/or frozen.

Improved Larabars

Makes about 16 bars

Unlike most of the variations available commercially, homemade bars offer the chance for using organic ingredients and crispy nuts. These bars taste almost like brownies! There are endless variations on flavors. You can try banana/walnut or cherry/coconut, lemon/pecan…the kids love to experiment with this recipe. Here is one of our favorites: chocolate/cherry with either almonds or walnuts.

1 cup chopped dates, pitted
1 cup other dried fruit or combination dried fruit (raisins, cherries, or figs)
1 1/2 tablespoons cocoa powder
Pinch or two salt
1 1/3 cups soaked and dehydrated nuts, such as almonds, walnuts, pecans
1/3 cup add-ins (shredded coconut, soaked and dehydrated seeds, chocolate shavings, mini chocolate chips)
Additional tablespoons of water, if needed

1. In a food processor, process dates, dried fruit, cocoa powder and salt until all is chopped up. It will be like a thick paste and may roll up into a ball. Move contents from food processor to a bowl.

2. Put nuts (and seeds or coconut, if desired) in the food processor. Process to a coarse meal.

3. Break up the fruit paste into chunks and add back to food processor. Add chocolate shavings or mini chips (if using). Process to incorporate all ingredients. It may roll up into a ball. Press with your finger—does it hold together? If not, add additional water, tablespoon by tablespoon.

4. Press the dough into an 8-inch or larger glass casserole dish. Refrigerate for 15 to 30 minutes until hardened enough to cut.

5. Remove from the fridge and cut into bars.

6. Store the pan of bars in the refrigerator, covered tightly so they don't dry out. Or wrap each bar individually and store in the refrigerator for an easy grab-and-go snack!

Goat Cheese Truffles

Makes about 20 servings

This is a delicious and protein-rich treat. And of course, the cheese is a cultured fermented food as is the raw cacao powder.

> **6 ounces fine-quality dark chocolate**
> **6 ounces chevre goat cheese**
> **2 tablespoons maple syrup (or honey)**
> **½ teaspoon vanilla extract**
> **½ teaspoon grated fresh ginger (optional)**
> **¼ cup raw cacao powder**

1. Melt chocolate in a glass bowl over a pan of barely simmering water. Stir until just melted.

2. Let the chocolate cool slightly.

3. In a bowl, mix together the goat cheese, maple syrup, vanilla, ginger until the mixture is well blended.

4. Whisk in the chocolate, cover the mixture, then chill for at least one hour or until it is firm.

5. Form heaping teaspoons of the mixture into balls and roll the balls into the cacao powder.

6. Chill the truffles on a plate or glass baking container for 30 minutes or until they are firm.

Popsicles

I love making small popsicles during the summer. I like the silicon reusuable containers from Tivoli (see page 131). But you can also use small paper cups with wooden popsicle sticks in a pinch.

> **Pickle brine (seriously good)**
> **Kraut brine**
> **Kefir with blended fruit**
> **Yogurt with blended fruit**
> **Fruit diluted with water**
> **Watermelon or melon juice**

1. Choose one ingredient from above and freeze for several hours.

2. Come up with your own! Be creative!

Easy Egg-Free Vanilla Pudding

This recipe is my modified version of Mark Bittman's Vanilla Pudding.
4 servings

Time: 20 minutes, plus chilling (but it tastes great warm too)

Puddings thickened with tapioca starch are dead easy—practically foolproof and fairly quick. Start with half-and-half or cream, or at least use whole milk.

2 1/2 cups whole organic milk (or half cream and half milk is richer)
1/3 cup organic sugar (or honey) or even less
Pinch salt
1 vanilla bean or 1 teaspoon vanilla extract
3 tablespoons organic tapioca starch
2 tablespoons unsalted organic butter, softened (optional but awesome)

1. Combine 2 cups of half-and-half or milk, sugar, and salt in a small or medium sauce pot. Place pot over medium-low heat. If using vanilla bean, split in half lengthwise and scrape seeds with a small, sharp knife into milk or half-and-half and, then add the pod. Cook just until mixture begins to steam.

2. Combine tapioca and remaining milk or half-and-half in a bowl and blend; there should be no lumps. Remove pod from pot and discard.

3. Add tapioca mixture. Cook, stirring occasionally, until mixture starts to thicken and before it barely reaches a boil–about 5 minutes.

4. Immediately reduce heat to very low and stir for another 5 minutes or so, until thick. Stir in butter and vanilla extract if desired.

5. Pour mixture into a quart-sized dish or 4 to 6 small bowls.

6. Serve warm or refrigerate until chilled. Pudding will thicken a bit in the fridge.

Variations

- Chocolate: Shave or finely chop 2 ounces bittersweet chocolate. Stir into pudding when adding the butter or add a few drops of peppermint extract with chocolate for a chocolate peppermint taste.
- Banana: Puree one banana and reduce sugar to 1/4 or less.
- Cinnamon: Add 1/8 teaspoon with step 1.

Healthiest and Easiest Fudge Ever

No cooking required! And super simple to make. What more can you ask for in a fudge recipe with healthy fats and nutrients?

Feel free to substitute ingredients with this recipe. Coconut oil works great, but raw butter is also amazing. I find that this combination of ingredients doesn't have a coconut oil taste. I use a food processor or my Blendtec, but you can use a hand mixer.

1/2 cup virgin coconut oil
1/2 cup dark chocolate chopped fine
1/3 cup raw honey or less
Dash salt
Dash cayenne pepper (optional, but you should try it!)
1/2 teaspoon vanilla

1. If the coconut oil is hard, you may want to heat it briefly to soften it a bit. I keep it at room temperature, but in the winter, I need to place the glass jar into some hot water to soften.

2. In a food processor, using the regular blade or a high-speed mixer, add all ingredients and blend until well combined.

3. Place parchment paper in a loaf pan and cover the bottom and sides of the pan, or you can oil up the bottom and sides with coconut oil.

4. Scrape your fudge "dough" into the pan, and fold the parchment paper over the top of the fudge.

5. Gently press down to even out the thickness of the fudge to be about 1/2 inch thick.

6. Take out the carefully wrapped fudge and place in the freezer or refrigerator until it has hardened. Or place entire pan in the freezer.

7. In the freezer, it takes about 20 to 30 minutes to harden.

8. Cut into small squares and enjoy!

Chocolate!

What to Look For: Chocolate geeks would say chocolate is pure—nothing else should be added. Period. But many would disagree. A few other ingredients can enhance the taste of chocolate and make it even more enjoyable. I consider the following to be perfectly fine additions: salt, nibs, spices such as chili, ginger, cinnamon, and real vanilla (not vanillin which is made from wood). Emulsifiers are certainly not necessary, and I try to avoid any soy-based ones.

Chocolate can be ethical and political

Cacao is grown within 20 degrees latitude of the equator so unless you live within that area, you are not purchasing local chocolate. As a Californian, my best choice is to purchase chocolate from a country that grows and makes its own. And after seeing the documentary The Dark Side of Chocolate, whch reveals slave child labor, and talking to Kallari (a farm cooperative and producer in Ecuador), I am more resolute in supporting fair-trade organic only, preferably beans not bars in the country of origin. You can watch the movie for free at:
documentaryheaven.com/the-dark-side-of-chocolate/#

Chocolate is a treat rather than a staple. I think you should get the most bang for your buck. And unfortunately, high quality is usually correlated to higher prices for this indulgence. But it's worth it!

How to choose chocolate

Read the ingredients! Eliminate bars with ingredients that are not healthy or whole. If you need to Google an ingredient, then it's probably best to put the bar back on the shelf. Look for fair trade and organic on the label. Bars that contain more than 75% of pure chocolate are higher in antioxidants (flavoinoids) and lower in sugar content.

I have researched several companies, so following are my top recommendations. The first three are all made within the actual country in which the beans are grown. All bars should be gluten free. Most of the following companies pay much higher prices than fair trade for their beans, so the quality and flavor of the beans will be seen in these amazing "happy" chocolates.

- **Grenada Chocolate**: Organic cooperative in Grenada. Amazing flavor. grenadachocolate.com
- **Pacari**: First biodynamic organic farm to bar cooperative in Ecuador pacarichocolate.com
- **Kallari**: Farmer-owned cooperative in Ecuador (kallarichocolate.com)
- **Rogue Chocolate**: Wild harvested from wild, rare cacao in Bolivia. Smooth and mellow chocolate. The Silvestre 75% bar is my favorite. roguechocolatier.com

❦ **Taza**: Organic, Mexican style chocolate using Oaxacan stone mills called molinos to grind the cacao. These stones minimally refine the cacao beans, capturing their vibrant flavors and allowing tiny bits of cacao and organic cane sugar to remain in the finished chocolate. tazachocolate.com

If you can't find great chocolate locally, then check out some the options that follow. Many of the companies listed have links for you to make purchases online. Another great online source is chocosphere.com. I am fortunate in having the Chocolate Garage (thechocolategarage.com) in Palo Alto, CA. Sunita, the owner, runs an intimate small shop of "happy" fair-trade, great tasting chocolate. She will ship group orders.

How to taste chocolate

Surprisingly, this process is similar to wine tasting, and serious chocolate nerds can get pretty intense when judging chocolate.

1. Make sure the chocolate is at room temperature. Like cold cheese, cold chocolate won't allow the scent and full flavors to come through.

2. Before you taste, look at your chocolate closely. You want chocolate that has a glossy surface and is free from blemishes. If the surface is scarred, cloudy, or gray, this may be a sign that the chocolate is old or has been subject to extremes in temperature or handling. Next, break the chocolate into pieces. You want a chocolate with a clean, hard "snap" to it. If it bends or crumbles, either the quality is low or the chocolate is old.

3. Good chocolate will smell strongly of chocolate. Rub your fingers over the surface to warm the chocolate, and then smell the bar. If it doesn't smell like chocolate, or if it smells primarily of vanilla or other added ingredients, it probably won't taste very much like chocolate either. Chocolate easily picks up odors from its environment, so be aware if your chocolate smells like coffee, tea, or other aromatic foodstuffs.

4. Finally, taste the chocolate. Pay attention to the way it melts in your mouth, and let it hit the roof of your palate. Does it feel waxy? Does it leave a slightly slippery feeling? Does it feel sandy or smooth? In general, a smooth, velvety feel is preferred.

5. Notice which flavors you can taste in the chocolate. Common descriptions of chocolate include floral, citrus, berry, coffee, and wine undertones. Notice if the flavor bursts out all at once or if it gradually builds in intensity and lingers after the chocolate is consumed. Above all, trust your own taste buds. Chocolate preference is very personal, and you know what tastes good to you. So, select chocolate that you will enjoy eating.

Appendix A: Equipment

These are some of my favorite kitchen tools. I find they make cooking easier and more enjoyable. However, it took me a while to figure out what works best for me, my family, and my classes. I certainly made some purchases that I regretted later. This was a journey of testing and planning before I could build my kitchen toolbox. I hope you find these as useful and durable as I have.

Links to these items are available on my amazon store through my website's home page, except for the Excalibur and Wise Choice Market. Visit my website at LisasCounterCulture.com if you want to see pictures, get more product details, or to place an order. I do receive a small affiliate commission if you purchase an item through my store. (Thank you in advance if you choose to do so.)

Pickl-It Jars: I do sell the Pickl-It jars locally in the California bay area. I am a value-added reseller, so when you purchase through my site, you receive support from me with troubleshooting or questions that may come up, as well as ideas on what to ferment. You can also order directly from Pickl-It (Pickl-It.com).

Juicers and Blenders: I did a blog post on comparing various juicers and high-speed blenders (Blendtec versus Vitamix) and you can find that on my website under Links.

Omega 8000 Juicer: It uses a single auger to extract juice. It is easy to assemble and, more importantly, easy and fast to clean. So easy that I use it daily. The juice is processed at a low rpm speed, so I get less friction and less heat, preserving the enzymes that can be destroyed by heat. The Omega 8000 also grinds boneless meat, makes nut butter, raw ice cream (basically feed frozen fruits through the juicer) and extrude pasta with the different nozzles that are included. I have not tried these applications yet.

Blendtec: Blends the heck out of anything! I like it better than others for several reasons but mostly because of its two-sided blade design. Stuff doesn't get stuck at the bottom of the jar as it dose with the traditional 4-sided blade jar—so no waste! I It's a great design—easy to move it out of the way to get everything out of the jar. And no **tamper**! Push the preprogrammed buttons and stand back while it sucked everything down to the blade.

Victorinox 10-Inch Chef's Knife: A great everyday knife that sells for about $30.

I have several and love them. Highly rated by *Cook's Illustrated* too! I even pack it when we travel!

Scanpan: A perfect pan for dosa and almost everything else. Safe, easy to clean and a lifetime guarantee.

Hamiliton Crockpot: This slow cooker is perfect for bone broth, whole chickens, pulled pork, short ribs and more. Lead free. I have the 8 quart size and find it perfect for making large batches of bone broth (primary reason I bought it).

Hydrofarm Seedling Heat Mat: Got icicles in your house? You need this mat to give those heat-loving ferments like dosa and dairy kefir some help. It warms the ferment to 15 to 20°F over room temperature. Good for starting seed germination too.

Excalibur 9-Tray Dehydrator: A great product for tons of applications. I'm always discovering new things to try with this dehydrator. Get the largest one that you can. It's easy to fill all the trays once your harvest comes in. You can even fit in a 1.5 Pickl-It when making yogurt. I prefer this brand instead of a stainless steel one since it regulates the temperature more accurately (metal conducts heat, so it's harder to keep steady) and dehydrating is done at low temps so there's no issue of leaching toxins into your food.

Swing Top Glass Bottle (1 Liter Italian): Perfect for bottling second ferments of water kefir, kombucha, ginger ale and beet kvass. Be sure to get Italian-made glass.

Spiral Slicer: I own the New and Essential Tri-Blade Spiral Vegetable Slicer. Add grain-free and healthy noodles into your diet. Zucchini noodles are the primary reason why I got this slicer, but I love making long strands of daikon for fermenting too. Great for many vegetables and fun for kids to use. Easy to clean. I tried a few other designs and brands and found this one to be the best.

Garlic Press: The all-stainless-steel Kuhn Rikon Garlic Press is another of *Cook's Illustrated's* highly recommended items. And I agree.

Food Scale: OXO Good Grips Food Scale is what I have. But most digital scales are inexpensive and reliable. Be sure there's a "tare" button to zero-out your scale, as well as the ability to weigh in ounces and grams.

Popicles: Orka 4-Ice Pops are small and twisted in shape, made of silicon so no weird plastic stuff on your food. Easy to clean and fun to use. I ended up buying two sets for pickles and kraut brine pickles!

Stainless Steel Stock Pot: I have three of these workhorses in my kitchen: a 4 quart, 8 quart and 16 quart. Great for brewing a gallon of kombucha. I use the large one to make some serious chicken bone broth.

Dutch Oven: I love using these for stews, braises and soups. I like Le Creuset, but there are other good brands to select from. I have several sizes. They are pricey, but they often go on sale, and you can also find Le Creuset store outlets.

Appendix B: Food Resources

Here are the sources that I believe are of the highest quality, sustainable and ethical. The farmers and ranchers listed here are working hard to provide humanely raised, pastured and sustainably farmed products. Wherever possible, I've tried to list them in the order that they are appear in this book.

Kombucha: Lisa's Kombucha Tea Blend is an organic fair trade loose ratio of green, white and black tea that keeps your scoby healthy and your kombucha tasty. I also like Mountain Rose Herbs (mountainroseherbs.com) for teas and herbs.

Cultures and Kefir Grains: Local and fresh are best. They are even better if you find a source that has properly cared for these products in anaerobic conditions. I do offer these cultures locally and will consider shipping too. Another option is to check your local Weston A. Price Chapter (westonaprice.org/local-chapters/find-local-chapter) for other sources.

Fermented Vegetables, Brines and Caldwell Starter:

Farmhouse Culture: farmhouseculture.com
This company is the only local organic kraut/kimchi producer that I know definitely uses the proper temperature and does ferment anaerobically. The cure time is at least three weeks, but if you ferment/cure for another week or so, it should be ready to eat. The brine is available at the farmer's market when there is extra (there tends to be more in the spring and summer than in the winter). Available at Whole Foods Markets, mail order and several bay area farmer's markets.

Wise Choice Market: wisechoicemarket.com (affiliate link is available on my website's home page) and hopefully available soon in local bay area stores.
This company offers a variety of properly fermented vegetables and brines that are made with organic ingredients and fermented for 12 weeks using the Caldwell starter. I prefer the taste of homemade but this is a great option for in between times and for traveling. Two day shipping during the week and shipped frozen.

Caldwell Starter: This is the only starter that I recommend. This is a broad spectrum starter, meticulously sourced from organic vegetables, not from a dairy source. wisechoicemarket.com (affiliate link is available on my website's home page).

Where to Get Real Milk: California has two licensed raw milk dairies: Claravale and Organic Pastures. Available in local health food stores and groceries (not Whole Foods). Bay area weekly delivery to drop points is available from realfoodbayarea.com. Both raw milk dairies offer cow milk. Claravale also offers goat milk.

Pasteurized Organic Cream Top Milk is available from Straus Creamery (also under the Trader Joe's Cream Top Whole Milk label) and from St. Benoit. See realmilk.com for other sources in the United States

Bay Area Sources for Animal Products Direct from the Farm

Old Creek Ranch: Family owned and located in Cayucos, CA. Beef, Lamb and Goat, organic pastured pork lard and chicken fat, and eggs are available.
Find them at farmer's markets or check out their website. oldcreekranch.net

Fiesta Farm: Pastured chicken (organs, feet and head) and eggs and soon turkeys! Offered at farmer's markets and through CSA shares (Community Supported Agriculture). Soy/corn free chickens and eggs are available. fiestafarm.net

Full of Life Farm: An Oregon farm that delivers to drop points in the bay area, Portland, and Oregon. Soy/corn-free beef, goat, lamb, pigs, turkeys, and chickens. Pastured and modeled after the Polyface farm. Bernard Smith, the owner, is raising these animals as nature intended with rotated pastures and natural food sources. fulloflifefarm.com

Evergreen Acres: Pastured soy and corn free duck eggs and other farm products. Email Jane Hulme at info@petstouch.com

Other Sources for Prepared Real Food

Red Boat Fish Sauce: The best! Find it on my amazon store from my website's home page. I stock it for local buyers. It has two ingredients, wild black anchovies and sea salt—that's it! Virgin press with nothing added—no water, sugar or MSG. Use it sparingly when converting your fish sauce recipes. I had to reduce the amount to half. The only commercial fish sauce fermented in wooden barrels for at least 11 months. redboatfishsauce.com

Grindstone Bakery: Gluten, dairy and yeast free traditional breads and cookies made by hand from milling the grains, soaking and a long natural fermentation. Available in the bay area and online at grindstonebakery.com

Three Stone Hearth: Prepared traditional foods are delivered throughout the bay area. Samples of their offerings include bone broth, rendered fats, kefir and more. Based on Weston A. Price principles. threestonehearth.com

Sigona's: Extra virgin olive oil and vinegars. Taste before you buy. Organic and harvest dates are provided. Shipping is available. sigonas.com

<u>Eat Wild</u>: Find a farmer near you. eatwild.com

<u>Local Harvest</u>: Find farmer's markets and farmers near you. localharvest.org

<u>Weston A. Price Foundation</u>: Find out about traditional diets and health. Their annual shopping guide is worth the membership price alone. wapf.org

<u>GAPS Diet</u>: Acronym for Gut and Psychology Syndrome. A digestive healing diet created by Dr. Natasha Campbell-McBride. Gapsdiet.com

Recipe Index